Cambridge History of Medicine

EDITORS: CHARLES WEBSTER and CHARLES ROSENBERG

Public health in Papua New Guinea

Public health in Papua New Guinea
Medical possibility and social constraint, 1884–1984

Donald Denoon
The Research School of Pacific Studies,
The Australian National University
with Kathleen Dugan and Leslie Marshall

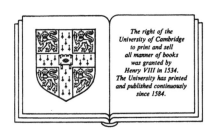

The right of the
University of Cambridge
to print and sell
all manner of books
was granted by
Henry VIII in 1534.
The University has printed
and published continuously
since 1584.

CAMBRIDGE UNIVERSITY PRESS
CAMBRIDGE

NEW YORK   NEW ROCHELLE   MELBOURNE   SYDNEY

PUBLISHED BY THE PRESS SYNDICATE OF THE UNIVERSITY OF CAMBRIDGE
The Pitt Building, Trumpington Street, Cambridge, United Kingdom

CAMBRIDGE UNIVERSITY PRESS
The Edinburgh Building, Cambridge CB2 2RU, UK
40 West 20th Street, New York NY 10011–4211, USA
477 Williamstown Road, Port Melbourne, VIC 3207, Australia
Ruiz de Alarcón 13, 28014 Madrid, Spain
Dock House, The Waterfront, Cape Town 8001, South Africa

http://www.cambridge.org

First published 1989
First paperback edition 2002

A catalogue record for this book is available from the British Library

Library of Congress Cataloguing in Publication data
Denoon, Donald
Public health in Papua New Guinea.
(Cambridge history of medicine)
Bibliography.
Includes index.
1. Public health – Papua New Guinea – History.
I. Dugan, Kathleen.
II. Marshall, Leslie B.
III. Title.
IV. Series.
RA558.P3D46   1989   362.1′0995′3   88-23749

ISBN 0 521 36030 7 hardback
ISBN 0 521 52302 8 paperback

Contents

Acknowledgements

The research was begun by Dr Leslie Marshall and Dr Kathy Dugan, interviewing elderly mission medical personnel. Their medical and scientific expertise produced a series of illuminating interviews, and provoked lively discussion on the scope and content of this enterprise. I much regret that the project had to be completed and written up without their assistance. The work does, however, reflect their enthusiasm and general direction, if not always their particular insights and expertise. Julie Gordon processed the words patiently and precisely. Win Mumford drafted the maps with care and flair. Trudi Tate brought order to anarchic references, and clarity to the text. Many scholars have been generous in their encouragement and criticism, most notably Barry Smith, Janice Reid, Jim Gillespie, Diane Langmore and Hank Nelson. The notes mainly list published academic works and medical reports and archival sources; but the analysis was powerfully advanced by many practising doctors, who were not only generous with their time and ideas, but also delightful subject to interview. The most important of these are Wilfred Moi, John Biddulph, B. G. Burton-Bradley, Peter Strang, Roy Scragg, Ian Maddocks, Robert Black, Tony Radford, Reia Taufa, Timothy Pyakalyia, and Quentin Riley. The most generous and scabrous, critical and self-critical, and most revealing of all the interview subjects was the late Sir John Gunther, to whose vivid memory this work is dedicated.

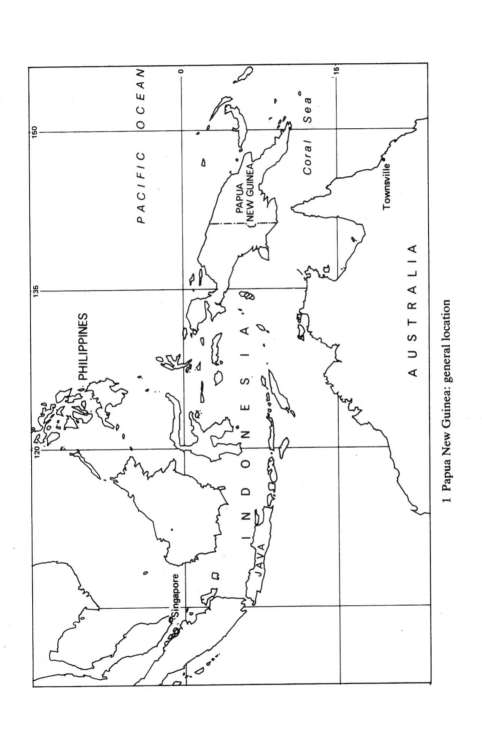

1 Papua New Guinea: general location

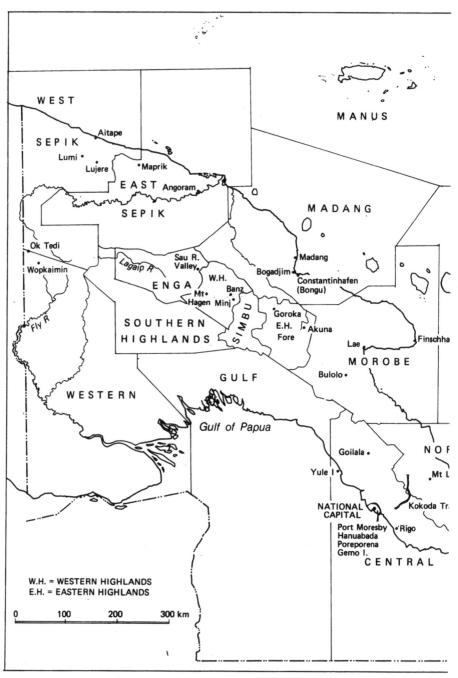

2 Papua New Guinea: provinces and place names

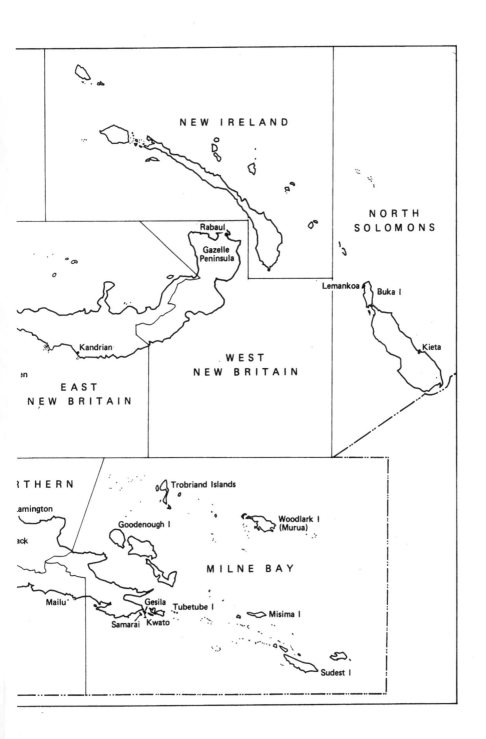

NEW IRELAND

NORTH
SOLOMONS

Rabaul

Gazelle
Peninsula

Lemankoa

Buka I

Kieta

Kandrian

WEST
NEW BRITAIN

EAST
NEW BRITAIN

an

THERN

amington

ack

Trobriand Islands

Woodlark I
(Murua)

Goodenough I

MILNE BAY

Mailu

Gesila

Samarai Kwato

Tubetube I

Misima I

Sudest I

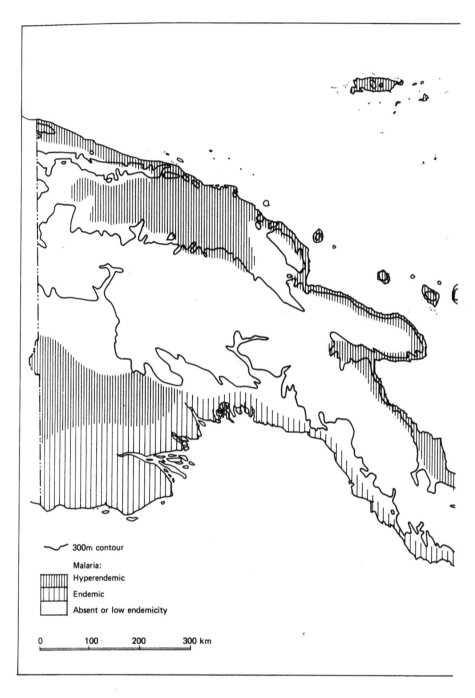

3 Papua New Guinea: physical conditions which influence disease distribution

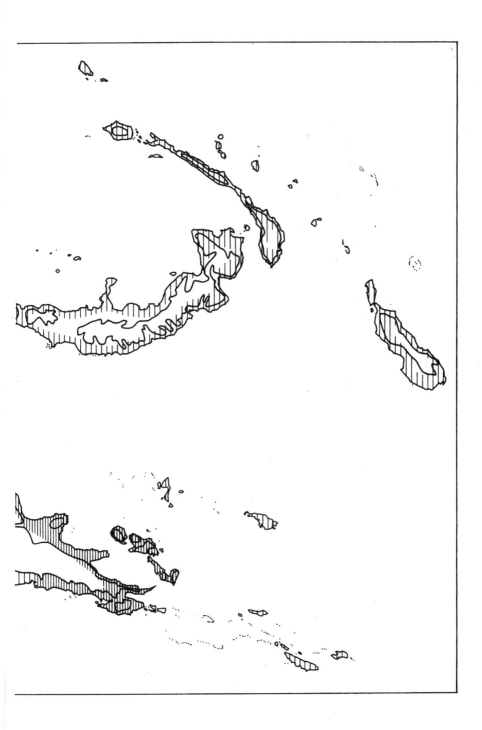

Introduction

The social study of medicine used to be inhibited by the awe which doctors inspired in lay people. Doctors would conduct their esoteric debates among themselves, confident that the leading issues were purely technical in nature. During the past generation, however, the caring professions have become less confident of their prescriptions, and correspondingly willing to discuss their concerns with a wider public. Meanwhile the soaring cost of medical services has provoked wider debate about health policies, and closer attention to the costs and benefits of programmes. The community as a whole now funds services which most individual patients cannot afford.

The new openness is especially marked in those regions roughly described as the 'third world', newly emancipated from colonial administrations. Colonial governments discouraged public debate on social policies generally, and consumers of those policies lacked a forum for canvassing their needs. Independence created forums for debate, and continuing poverty and low standards of living promoted discussion of the relative merits of health programmes as against education, or agricultural extension, or any other element of 'development'. These discussions have also been internationalised, to match the international implications of any single country's health hazards. The present AIDS epidemic and the remarkable revival of malaria are only the most visible of many concerns which agitate researchers, practitioners and planners throughout the world.

The burgeoning of social studies of medicine during the past decade has opened many useful lines of enquiry for us: nevertheless there are peculiar features which determine the scope of the present enquiry. Perhaps the most peculiar feature is the amorphous nature of our subject matter. Doctors and nurses aspire to promote health, the most diffuse and indefinable of human conditions. We usually value our well-being only when it is impaired, and then each person places a different value on pain, distress and disease. The caring professions do not create a measurable product (though they certainly generate statistics). Nor do they create good health: as a rule they treat specific kinds of illness. The influence of medical workers may be profound, but it cannot be measured accurately.

This observation forced us to abandon our bold intention to study the changing health status of the people of Papua New Guinea. That retreat is justified also by the immense variety of health conditions throughout the country. In the 1980s, some communities enjoy levels of health and

1

nutrition which are the envy of most of the world; while other communities
– usually remote from markets and services – endure appalling privations
and high levels of morbidity and mortality. To lump everyone together
might produce an average which no single community experiences: it would
also obliterate those differences from region to region, between town and
country, and between men and women, which should properly be high-
lighted. From time to time we describe the health status of particular
communities; but these accounts are all tentative, and their purpose is to
illustrate the problems which doctors and nurses observed and confronted.

The subject matter precludes a study of public health, but it does
provide the evidence for examining the caring professions. Although we
cannot confidently measure their influence on general health, we can
certainly evaluate their impact on public health policy and programmes.
Since the 1890s, doctors have largely determined health policy, subject to
very little constraint. Until the 1910s, the colonial state in New Guinea and
in Papua was too sickly to resist medical advice. In the 1920s an attempt was
made to impose planters' interests on the Department of Health in New
Guinea; but the medical authorities brushed aside this intrusion into their
professional autonomy. During the 1950s it suited the Public Health
Department of the amalgamated territories to pretend that it was obeying
instructions from the Australian government; but policies were actually
proposed and implemented by doctors. On the eve of Independence (in
1975), officers of the department and representatives of the mission services
integrated their institutions, and framed health policies for the endorsement
of the new democratic government. From time to time doctors have
genuinely attempted to involve lay people in the formulation of policy, and
in its implementation: yet doctors have always had science on their side, and
lay people have been reluctant to interfere. Responsibility for health policy
has therefore been much more clearly defined than any other part of
policy-formulation.

Though doctors have been self-consciously the instruments of western
science, they have obeyed a most flexible and accommodating master.
Policy has always been justified by science, but that statement tells us rather
little about the source of policy ideas. To anticipate the argument of the
body of this book, medical planners have been guided by continually
changing perceptions, and those perceptions are only partly 'scientific':
social perceptions are equally significant.

A decisive influence on policy has been the state of medical knowledge: doctors and nurses are naturally most interested in conditions which
will respond to treatment or yield to preventive measures, and least
interested in conditions which seem likely to endure. New therapeutic
possibilities have often persuaded medical authorities to devote their
attention and resources to previously tolerated suffering. Quinine focused
interest on malaria, arsenicals excited interest in yaws, and BCG provoked
a campaign to eradicate tuberculosis. Although New Guinea and Papua

were among the most remote provinces of western medicine, doctors quickly learned about new therapies, and could implement new therapeutic regimes very swiftly.

If therapeutic possibility were the only influence on medical perceptions, this would be a very short monograph; but social possibility is as important as technical opportunity, in shaping perceptions and programmes. The first half of the study deals with the era of 'tropical medicine', a body of theory and practice which influenced practitioners in tropical regions from the turn of this century until about the 1940s. Stated simply, that body of theory assumed that health status was largely determined by physical environment. There were distinct tropical diseases which were mainly untreatable. From this starting point, doctors were disposed to treat only those few conditions which would respond to treatment, and to concentrate their efforts on the protection of enclaves of 'temperate' settlers and their labourers from the consequences of living in a tropical environment. General improvements in living standards seemed impossible, but quarantine and racial segregation might create a few safe environments for key personnel. The mood of medical planners was usually pessimistic and defensive, and their programmes reflected their pessimism. The second half of the study begins with the Pacific War, and the adoption of remarkable new drugs – the 'magic bullets' – which inspired heroic offensives against specific killer diseases during the 1950s. These campaigns marked a decisive shift from defence to resolute attack and the optimism survived the limited success of the campaigns themselves. Then as euphoria dwindled, medical planners grasped the new strategic vision of 'primary health care', an era which began in the 1950s and is still with us. Again stated simply, the theories brought together under this attractive rubric assumed that the whole population could, and should, enjoy better living conditions and longer life. That vision was more appropriate to democratic independence than to autocratic colonialism, and it implied not only an equalising of access to services throughout the population, but also some involvement of free and responsible citizens in the formulation and implementation of programmes. At first sight, therefore, 'primary health care' seems diametrically opposed to the earlier vision of 'tropical medicine': optimistic, participatory and egalitarian, where the earlier strategy had been defensive, authoritarian and divisive. Yet the two approaches share some features in common, most notably the fact that each is a strategic vision devised by medical workers and presented to the general population for endorsement rather than discussion. Primary health care is a *doctors'* vision of public health, and its adoption does not alter the fact that health policy remains a matter of doctors' dilemmas.

As a case study, Papua New Guinea presents a number of unusual features which need to be remembered if comparisons are drawn with other countries. The eastern half of the island of New Guinea, together with the islands to the north and east, are compact in size but varied in ecology. The territory is well within the tropics (from 2°S to 10°S), but the environment varies from steamy lowlands to crisp highlands ranging above 3,000 metres. The present population is small (about three million people), but culturally and economically diverse. In the nineteenth century the people chose to live in such small and self-contained communities that something like 700 distinct languages evolved; and their precarious well-being was largely the consequence of their isolation from each other and the rest of the world. Partly because of health hazards, but also through the country's isolation from major trade routes, colonisation was relatively late. Only in 1884 did Germany annexe New Guinea, while Britain declared a protectorate over British New Guinea (soon re-named Papua). The country is divided from Australia by the narrow and shallow Torres Strait, so Australia became (and remains) the dominant external power. The new Commonwealth of Australia succeeded Great Britain as the colonial authority in Papua in 1906, and conquered the German garrison in New Guinea in 1914, retaining that territory under a League of Nations Mandate. After the Japanese invasion of 1942, New Guinea and Papua were amalgamated administratively in 1945, and became independent in 1975.

Colonialism was not only late, but also perfunctory. The densely populated highlands were explored only in the 1920s and 1930s, and regularly administered after the Pacific War: many people could boast that they remembered the arrival of the Australians when they formally withdrew 30 years later. One consequence of this dilatoriness was that economic development was slow. The early colonial economy was based squarely upon copra, supplemented by gold in the 1890s and especially during the 1930s. Since the 1960s the cash economy has diversified into coffee and cocoa, while large mining enclave projects export copper and some silver and gold. However, social services did not wait upon the growth of the colonial economy. Since the 1950s, high levels of Australian aid have enabled the government to provide a wider range of social services than the colonial economy could sustain on its own. Among the most impressive of these services was the Public Health Department, which first supplemented and later incorporated the work of medical missions, integrating them all into a single national health care system by the time of Independence. Medical programmes have scarcely been constrained by finance: a more serious obstacle has been the difficulty of attracting or training sufficient doctors and nurses to realise the ambitious visions of health planners.

Medical authorities enjoyed an autonomy from the colonial state, which may be unusual. The administration was implemented by a variety of technical departments, each of which looked to its Australian counterpart and was only loosely coordinated with other branches of the local administration. Among the specialist departments, Public Health enjoyed remarkable eminence, employing almost all the graduate workers in the country, deploying a large proportion of the financial resources, and claiming the greatest ability to transform lives. The medical authorities took advantage of a narrow enthusiasm for technique which influenced all branches of government, and enouraged the view that each department must be the best judge of its own programmes. Only with the advent of self-government and Independence were the departments firmly subordinated to coordination and political control.

Independence did not decisively change the status of health workers. Many experienced medical administrators left the country, but they were replaced by indigenous doctors, and the department preserved the tradition that senior medical administrators must possess medical qualifications. Since Independence was late and amicable, colonial administrators enjoyed an Indian summer which was denied their counterparts in Africa and Asia; and the independent government felt no need to revolutionise the structures which it inherited.

In most dimensions, the present regime of public health in Papua New Guinea is remarkable: the population enjoys better access to more impressive services than most other parts of the 'third world', and any criticism of those services must be tempered by that perception. Medical authorities successfully anticipated Independence, so that the elected government inherited a more integrated, more responsive public health system than the colonial state enjoyed. At first sight this may seem to vindicate the strategy of primary health care. In the body of the book, however, we suggest that the rising living standards and increasing access of Papua New Guineans cannot be explained by the adoption of this new strategy. We also suggest that further advances in public health may require precisely the public involvement in policy and programmes which 'primary health care' proposed but cannot achieve.

We hope that the present work will add to an understanding of Papua New Guinea's particular experience; but we also hope to promote wider understanding and discussion of medical institutions generally. From the 1890s until the 1940s, medical authorities neglected many strategies for promoting the people's health; thereafter they grasped many of the opportunities which evolved technology presented; and increasingly they have construed good health as a goal which requires popular knowledge and enthusiastic participation as well as sophisticated drugs and techniques. Our purpose is to reinforce that perception, by demonstrating that health is not simply a series of doctors' dilemmas but – as a matter of life and death – a proper subject for universal concern and popular participation.

I
The rise and fall of tropical medicine

1
Pre-colonial health and disease

The context of this enquiry is the health of the people of Papua New Guinea, and its transformation over time. Regrettably, health is largely a subjective condition – 'well-being' is how we actually experience it: a contented condition which includes the absence of infection but is also a positive state. A study of health therefore cannot proceed directly: instead it relies upon inference. One source of evidence is the behaviour and observations of medical specialists, who are essentially experts in 'ill-being' rather than health itself. To compound the problem, we know very little about those specialists in pre-colonial Papua New Guinea. A recent review confesses that 'next to nothing is known empirically about the medical botany of Papua New Guinea. Even less is known about the full diagnostic and treatment regimes available traditionally.'[1]

In order to establish some base-line for this study, therefore, we have to make even more tenuous inferences from the physical environment. Since the physical environment itself changes, and human beings both change it and adapt to it,[2] this overview cannot pretend to completeness. Such evidence as we possess is best considered as the dozen surviving pieces of a vast jigsaw puzzle: they can only suggest the scale and tone of the whole picture.

The outline of New Guinea's environmental history is now fairly clear.[3] About 10,000 years ago, as the most recent ice-age receded and released water to swell the oceans, Torres Strait was submerged, separating New Guinea from the Australian continent, and stretching the intervals between the islands of the western Pacific. The gradual increase in temperature melted the last ice-sheets in the New Guinea highlands, leaving tropical rainforest as the most common vegetation pattern in areas not disturbed by human settlement. The hunters and gatherers stranded by this process found themselves isolated from changes everywhere else.

These small groups may have enjoyed quite good health:

> Like other nomadic peoples, these first small groups ... were probably free from many communicable diseases – for the reason that the sick, being unable to keep up, would be discarded, sanitation problems would be left behind, and the size of the groups would be insufficient to sustain acute infectious diseases.[4]

A rich variety of flora could yield a good living for these nomadic groups. From the point of view of nutrition, their chief difficulty may have been a shortage of protein. Along the coasts, and on small islands, fish and shell-fish provided ample protein, except when storms prevented fishing and collecting. Inland, protein was more problematic: bats, birds, lizards, snakes and marsupials could be caught, but there were no larger indigenous fauna, and only pigs and dogs (of the animals which could be domesticated) were available.[5] It could also be suggested that a handful of people, living off the land, must have been vulnerable to any climatic change, any natural disaster, or any chance infection which interrupted the daily tasks of collecting food.[6]

However, agriculture evolved in New Guinea relatively early – perhaps as much as 8,000 years ago – with far-reaching consequences for the environment. Some forest was destroyed by fire in hunting, but patches (and sometimes more than patches) were also cleared for swidden cultivation. While taro, yams, sago and bananas contributed to a large and reliable supply of bulk food, the shrinking forests of the upland interior offered less scope for bird and animal life: increased production of carbohydrate was purchased at the cost of diminished protein, except in pigs.[7] A denser human population became a decisive agent in the evolution of the landscape.

The transition to agriculture was uneven. A few scattered communities persisted in hunting and collecting their food into the twentieth century.[8] Along the coasts and on the smaller islands, fish and shellfish remain important to the present day, supplementing food crops. Even in the relatively dense highland populations, hunting game and collecting uncultivated foods provide a significant proportion of the diet. These circumstances generated a settlement pattern which profoundly affected the health status of small communities because of their relative isolation.

The degree to which communities were isolated from each other startled European observers from the nineteenth century onwards. It is possible that, in their surprise, commentators exaggerated somewhat in their accounts of the isolation they observed, and it is also possible that old trading networks were dissolved in the early colonial period, thus increasing the communities' isolation at that time.[9] At all events, it would be hard to find any other human population in excess of a million souls, which sustained so many mutually incomprehensible languages, so many named societies of small size, or such a thin tradition of exchanging specialist produce.[10]

The isolation of each Papua New Guinea community from most others (a condition commonly buttressed by warfare) was compounded by the isolation of the whole geographical area from sustained contact with the outside world. There were occasional visits by bird of paradise hunters and slave hunters from the islands to the west of New Guinea;[11] but these visitors were rare. The voyages of Europeans during the great age of discovery had surprisingly few consequences. As early as 1608 a Spanish fleet sailed through Torres Strait and fought with Mailu islanders near the 'tail' of Papua, but the profits of this encounter (some mats, some vegetables, and a handful of captives who were shipped out to Manila) were presumably too small to justify further voyages.[12] Until the last third of the nineteenth century, the paucity of trade goods, the ferocity of the inhabitants, and the prevalence of malaria, combined to construct a very effective *cordon sanitaire* around western Melanesia.[13] There were few occasions for exotic infections to enter the region; and those infections could touch only small populations, suppressing the possibility of their becoming endemic.

Epidemiologists suggest that such isolation allows certain deductions about patterns of health and illness. It is helpful first to distinguish between endemic and epidemic infections:

> Most infections do not lead to overt disease but only to sub-clinical infections that also confer immunity ... [Therefore we may distinguish] those that persist in a population over a long period of time, maintaining themselves in either human or non-human hosts [and which] are referred to as endemic ... They are characterised by high incidence and low morbidity, frequently due to the large number of subclinical infections that confer natural immunity. Such infections tend to survive well in small isolated populations as they do not normally kill their hosts.
>
> [Then there are those] infections that produce only acute symptomatic disease and generally have no reservoir other than man [and these] are referred to as epidemic ... In isolated groups they tend to have a high incidence, high morbidity, and high mortality. Such diseases generally 'burn out' quickly after introduction, because a large population is needed to supply new groups of susceptibles as those previously affected either die or become immune.[14]

The kinds of benefits conferred by this remoteness are well considered by Maddocks. He proposed that the earliest inhabitants

> disturbed few established ecosystems which in other parts of the world led to diseases such as trypanosomiasis [sleeping sickness], schistosomiasis [bilharzia] or leishmaniasis [dum-dum fever] [all of which rely upon the presence of a specific vector]. Scrub typhus provides a good local example of such an ecosystem, and it is one which the New Guinean came to fit into with relative comfort, rarely suffering from clinical disease compared to the [Pacific War soldier] who in war shattered the balance of rickettsia, mite, rodent and forest, to his acute disadvantage.[15]

To this already impressive list of absentees, Maddocks adds the acute crowd infections – measles, mumps, smallpox, chickenpox, rubella and the common cold – which required large population reservoirs.

Before we turn to endemic infections, we need to make one further distinction, to reflect three quite different styles of living which had evolved by the nineteenth century (see map 3). Along the coasts, and on the small islands, communities combined the gathering of shellfish with hunting and fishing, to yield protein: the cultivation of bananas, taro, yams and sago rounded out a good diet. Trading expeditions along the coast permitted some specialisation, such as the *hiri* trade on the south coast of Papua, which shipped thousands of pots west to the Gulf, to be exchanged for tons of sago and great logs for canoes.[16] By these means, population could exceed the carrying capacity of the immediate environment. The settlement pattern included villages of as many as several hundred people, living on the coast or in stilted dwellings perched over the water.

Behind the coasts, between the sea and the highlands, living conditions were less favourable. In this environment, population was sparse, cultivation was ill-developed, and there were also small bands of people who persisted in hunting and collecting their food. One of these small groups – the Wopkaimin – were surveyed by a team of medical researchers in 1983, during the development of the Ok Tedi gold mine nearby in the North Fly region. The preliminary observations described 720 people who

> live in scattered hamlets in a remote and mountainous region of dense bush and very high rainfall, at moderate altitudes. ... [T]he preliminary results show a very high crude infant mortality rate of 229 per 1000, low life expectancy, hyperendemic malaria, and widespread respiratory and skin disease.[17]

Nomadism and elusiveness – rather than sheer numbers – provided some defence against attack. In the highlands proper, elaborate agricultural systems sometimes evolved, especially during the past two or three hundred years when sweet potato could replace taro as a carbohydrate staple.[18] The settlement pattern usually consisted of hamlets, each with a men's house set about by smaller houses for women, children and pigs, and each located on high ground (such as a ridge top) commanding all possible approaches.

Probably the most widespread endemic infection was yaws. Almost universal in the lowlands, it was less common in the highlands. It is both debilitating and highly visible (as the flesh is slowly eaten away), but it is rarely fatal, so it was well adapted to survive even in very small populations. While treponemal infections became rare in early modern Europe, and survived only in a venereal form, the style of living among Melanesians – frequent physical contact among adults and children – permitted non-venereal yaws to persist. A happy consequence was the cross-immunity of the people to venereal syphilis.[19] Some herpes viruses almost certainly were endemic, for the same sorts of reasons.[20]

Malaria was also endemic in most of the country, apart from a few small enclaves, and with the important exception of the highlands. As recent developments have shown, there is no strictly environmental reason why malaria did not blanket the highlands as well as the lowlands. Anopheles mosquitoes inhabited the highlands,[21] but without infected humans to act as a reservoir, the mosquitoes did not transmit malaria. During the twentieth century, when malaria spread into the higher reaches of the Markham valley, it provoked the debilitating symptom of grossly enlarged spleens, like permanent pregnancy, which suggests the appalling effect which malaria might have on a fresh human population.[22] If (as seems possible) the highlands had relatively fast population growth rates and surplus populations were squeezed out to the foothills where malaria lay in wait, we may have part of the explanation for the relatively poor health observed throughout the highland fringe.[23] In coastal regions, on the other hand, many generations of exposure enabled people to suffer malaria as a low-grade endemic infection. Filariasis (or elephantiasis) which has the same mode of transmission as malaria, was also endemic to much of the country.[24]

As if yaws, filariasis and malaria were not enough to make life uncomfortable, tinea imbricata – an itchy skin infection – was widespread wherever a hot, sticky climate combined with close physical contact between infants and many adults. Tinea scarcely merits inclusion as a 'disease' as it is superficial in its effects, but it is a most irritating affliction which must have depressed those who suffered from it.[25]

The most notable killing infections were probably not the endemic ones, nor occasional exogenous diseases, but outbreaks of pneumonia and dysentery. In early colonial times, pneumococcal infections cut terrible swathes through Melanesian populations,[26] and it would be remarkable if these were the first outbreaks. The close living conditions of coastal villages, and especially of highlands hamlets, encouraged rapid transmission of any epidemic. Similarly, the rather casual approach towards personal hygiene makes it likely that amoebic dysentery occurred from time to time, no doubt affecting infants more drastically than adults.[27] On the other hand, bacterial varieties of dysentery were apparently unknown, and early colonial observers recorded quite elaborate latrines in some areas;[28] so we can only speculate on the frequency and intensity of these epidemics.

Some infections cannot be traced (or dismissed) in pre-colonial New Guinea with any degree of confidence. There seem to have been cases of leprosy before the end of the nineteenth century, but the relative isolation of one group from another, and the need for sustained and close contact for transmission, may explain the limited progress of the disease through the land.[29] Again, smallpox may have been brought in occasionally along the north coast, in the late nineteenth century and possibly earlier;[30] but if that did occur, then the isolation of the communities prevented it becoming endemic. Tuberculosis may not have occurred at all, prior to colonial times; but if it did, then it certainly made little progress into the region.[31]

How did people cope with these various afflictions? There is a burgeoning literature on the subject of Melanesian ethno-medicine, but much of it would endorse B.M. du Toit's report from the Akuna society in the eastern highlands:

In general Akunans did not utilize any great number or variety of plants. This seems to be in keeping with the general picture we have for Melanesians . . . While a variety of medications were known, they also lacked the magical and ritual complexity in preparation and administration found elsewhere, as in Africa. The poultice might be made, a leaf crushed and rubbed into or placed over a wound, a piece of bark chewed but that was the limit in most cases. [A specialist] however, due to particular powers which entered her at the time of her calling, can also remove the cause of discomfort by extracting it with some visible object.[32]

The close observation of animals, and experience in treating war wounds[33] provided many people with a sound grasp of basic anatomy. In some areas – notably parts of Enga in the far western highlands – surgical skill was refined for dealing with war wounds.[34] However, ethno-medicine (an indigenous body of knowledge re-tested and supplemented by specialists over the generations) was relatively undeveloped. Du Toit described the selection of a specialist among the Akuna. The novice was self-selected, when her predecessor felt too old to continue:

> Such a novice would now receive advice on medication and technique ... while also innovating her own forms of treatment. Payment would be made to a practitioner for services performed ... It seems that we are here dealing with the embryonic form of specialisation. While the [practitioner] still worked her gardens and still got married, she was the closest Akuna came to having a traditional full-time specialist.[35]

The circumstances of small, agrarian and uncentralised societies worked against the emergence of a special caste of medical (or any other) specialists. In consequence, many of the individuals mentioned in the literature are more properly described as shamans or sorcerers, called upon in medical emergencies to be sure, but schooled in psychic rather than clinical skills. A recent survey of therapies in the western highlands suggests that people attached very little importance to *materia medica*, and relied (with some confidence) on good nutrition to resist infection.[36]

We need not condescend towards the sorcery which Melanesians deployed in times of adversity. European medical practice in the nineteenth century was little better, and F.B. Smith concludes his study of *The people's health* with the judgment that the rise of the medical profession owed more to the doctor's shaman role as explainer of misfortune, than to his ability to heal the sick.[37] Comparing and contrasting western and indigenous therapies in a Sepik community in the twentieth century, Mitchell concludes that the coexistence of the two approaches is both natural and beneficial:

> As Christians readily turn to thought about God, Who both gives and takes away life, and appeal to Him to perform a healing miracle when sickness threatens life, so do the Lujere find explanatory comfort in their beliefs, centuries old, that promise surcease from suffering by the extraordinary powers of a witch's hand.[38]

Explanatory comfort is one thing, but health is another; and Melanesian beliefs and sorcerers were no better equipped than western doctors in the nineteenth century to encompass health. One series of incidents, well recorded in the 1950s and 1960s, illustrates significant features of the Melanesian predicament. During the 1950s, portions of the Fore people in the eastern highlands were severely afflicted by a 'laughing disease' which was unprecedented either in Fore experience, or indeed anywhere else in the world. As it attacked the central nervous system of the patient, she (or less commonly, he) steadily lost control of motor functions, and died through rolling into a fire, or falling from a steep path. If she survived these risks, she starved to death as the digestive system failed.[39] It required inter-disciplinary research in medical and social science, and the application of Nobel-quality intelligence, to unravel the aetiology of the disease. The eventual explanation for *kuru* forces us to believe in a virus which came into being among the Fore by chance, which can survive for many years before manifesting itself, and which is not transmitted by common social procedures. Even when western scientists established the nature of the disease, and its transmission, they were unable to cure sufferers.

The Fore people themselves sought explanation (and by implication a cure) in sorcery.[40] Rather than eliminating the affliction, sorcery seems to have exacerbated social tensions. What the *kuru* tragedy suggests is that 'ethno-medicine' had a very limited range of medications, and is better described as ethno-psychiatry. Confronted by a quite new disease, the community's first and overwhelming response was to seek a social rather than a scientific explanation: precisely the dominant response in western societies to the emergence of AIDS.

In the villages of the coast and islands, early Europeans considered that the villagers were able to cope with the endemic infections which were their lot.[41] What alarmed these visitors was the vulnerability of the village populations to infections brought in from abroad, rather than the debilitating effect of infections which persisted. Some optimists even hoped that health might be improved by colonialism:

> The well-drained lands of the Territory, where the plantation industries and other settlements are taking place, will be found to be quite as healthy as places such as Java, the Malay States and Ceylon, where better living conditions are attained.[42]

Events would falsify that prediction, but the writers may have been correct in identifying sanitation and clean water as the key to health status.

The generally cheerful picture which these observers painted should be treated with some caution. Garruto points to some circumstances which could generate false optimism: infanticide could take away infants with obvious physical defects; overt chronic cases were rare, because so few Melanesians lived to old age; and the absence of severe late-onset infection was partly a consequence of endemic early-onset disease. On this view, the non-survival of the sick or the deformed might create far too cheerful an impression: a sound health service is one which enables the sick and deformed to survive.[43] At least one of the early medical observers in Papua was shielded in this way, from a full appreciation of the complete health record. And as late as 1978, a WHO study of the North Fly region was puzzled by the good health and short life of the communities they surveyed.[44]

The small bands of nomads who inhabited the lands between the coasts and the highlands seem to have suffered the worst of both worlds. They did not enjoy the coastal people's easy access to protein, nor the highlanders' isolation from malaria. Morbidity and mortality rates were high, and would remain high even when improvement was recorded elsewhere.[45] In their anxiety to protect and nurture their young (and especially their young men) they sometimes adopted practices which were likely to be self-defeating.[46] It is in this region, too, that poor diet had its most striking ill-effects, for instance in goitre and endemic cretinism.[47]

For the pre-colonial highlands, due to the very late 'opening-up' of that region, we have good medical observations. Dr Heydon, of the Sydney School of Public Health and Tropical Medicine, visited the Mt Hagen area in 1934 – 35. He knew the coastal environment well, and was struck by the contrast between coastal and highland conditions. On the coast, heavy rainfall was merely a nuisance: in the highlands it was worse than that. Furthermore

> the climate is . . . often decidedly chilly. The natives wear no clothing which is protective against cold or rain and when necessary endure it stoically, standing for hours in wind and rain in a characteristic attitude, arms folded high up. The women, but not the men, commonly carry Karuka mats (made from Pandanus leaves) under which they squat on the ground if caught in the rain.
>
> Within their huts . . . the natives avoid the cold by means of a fire and the presence of several human beings and pigs within a confined space; there is no ventilation except the grass thatched roof through which the smoke slowly seeps.

The diet seemed superior to that of the coastal region: tuberculosis and dysentery, which had infested the coastal areas, were absent or insignificant and the burden of hookworm was decidedly lighter. These circumstances led Heydon to admire this 'healthy, well-nourished and cheerful race'.[48]

In one large area of medical practice, however, Melanesian societies seem not to have coped successfully at all. Nowhere were midwifery skills developed to compare with those which had evolved by the nineteenth century in most of the world.

> Papua New Guinea is unique in having numerous societies in which the role of the [traditional birth attendant] is non-existent, i.e. women normally deliver their babies alone or with the aid of a female relative who has no specific training in childbirth. In other areas, an elder woman with considerable experience is called in only if the delivery appears troublesome.[49]

The consequences of this included a very high maternal mortality rate, estimated variously at 30 or more maternal deaths for every thousand births.[50] Infant mortality was also very high, sometimes exceeding 300 deaths per thousand births, by the age of one year.[51] Since more boys than girls were born, and boys often enjoyed more attentive child-care, there was, a high proportion of males in all Melanesian societies. In recent times, Melanesia is the most masculine region in the world, with 108 males to every 100 females; and this is probably not a new circumstance.[52] A child who survived birth and early infancy had then to run the gauntlet of weaning from mother's milk to the bulky staple foods which made up all Melanesian adult diets, probably the most risky transition of any person's lifetime, as the digestive system was required to cope with a quite new quality and quantity of food.[53] These conditions add up to a population structure which is typical for what is now blandly called a 'developing country': high fertility rates, compensating for very high infant mortality, and the great majority at any time aged between 10 and 40.[54] If gender curves could be constructed, they would reveal that each cohort in these young populations comprised a majority of males.

In meeting most of the crises of daily life, neither household remedies nor specialist treatment made much difference to gross population figures, though they undoubtedly offered assurance and confidence. The well-being of Melanesians in the nineteenth century was not quite as impressive as early colonial observers believed; nor was it evenly distributed between the coastal villages, the inland foragers, and the highland hamlets. Those reservations aside, Melanesians did enjoy at least adequate health, and sometimes good health and good spirits. The predominant reason for this state of affairs was isolation: not only the isolation of the region from the rest of the world, but equally the isolation of each fairly small community from its neighbours. So long as that insularity remained intact, all infections and misfortunes were manageable, but the well-being of the population was fragile, and would be severely threatened by the increased interaction of people which the colonial era would necessarily involve.

2
The administration of
public health

Public health institutions and practices were initiated in Papua New Guinea late in the nineteenth century. They were an integral element of the colonial state, and the administrators were instruments of German and British empires which had developed fairly clear ideas about the proper regulation of public health. By the turn of the century these imperial ideas included a distinct body of theory about the administration of health services in the tropics.[1] There was little latitude for adapting ideas and practices to local circumstances, and the instituting of public health measures in Papua New Guinea is best understood as a local manifestation of a world-wide movement. In order to grasp the nature and purpose of these introduced services, we must digress to describe the perceptions and prescriptions which animated them.

Until the middle of the nineteenth century, western medicine had no particular advantage over the medical beliefs and practices of many other societies. Western medicine was an assemblage of techniques (especially surgical procedures) tested over time by an immense variety of university-taught or self-taught practitioners, having some scientific basis but no unifying scientific theory. The significant advances in public health of the early nineteenth century in Europe were mainly the product of bureaucratic control over clean water, sewage, and pure food and drink.[2] Medical practitioners operated in a legal limbo: sick individuals were free to consult whomsoever they pleased; anyone could advance a claim to be consulted. This unregulated condition persisted, in part, because there was no reliable way of distinguishing 'proper' treatments from dangerous ones, so long as they were all the product of empirical observation and personal intuition.

The foundation of modern medicine was laid only in the 1860s, with the discovery and elaboration of germ theory, a solid scientific structure on which many particular research findings could be raised. For our present purposes, the significance of that breakthrough is the professional organisation which it made possible. During the last third of the nineteenth century, professional associations of doctors formed throughout Europe, and in European colonies such as Australia. These associations were now able to distinguish between correct and improper treatments, and between 'real' doctors (who had graduated from universities) and 'quacks' (who had not). They were also emboldened to advise governments on matters of public policy.

Since Australia would become the source of much of the medical theory transplanted to Papua New Guinea, the rapid evolution of the medical profession in the Australian colonies may be instructive in this context.[3] By the end of the nineteenth century, the doctors in each of the colonies had joined into associations, which affiliated to the British Medical Association. Doctors used these associations to press recommendations upon the colonial governments, and in the process they built an exclusive registration procedure which barred 'quacks' from participation, which subordinated nurses and midwives as ancillary to doctors, and which marginalised other therapists such as opticians and dentists. As in Europe, so in Australia: doctors scrambled out of the ranks of the skilled working class and – as proper professional men – took their place beside lawyers in the ranks of the comfortable middle classes.

The swift progress of the medical profession coincided with an increasing concern on the part of colonial governments, to intervene in matters of public health which had previously been left to private initiative. In the Australian situation, it was often exogenous epidemics which provoked government action,[4] but governments went beyond the mere enactment of quarantine measures and the construction of isolation hospitals, to consider pure food, clean water, and slum clearance. Hospitals were still built largely by private subscription, but were increasingly subsidised by public moneys. Universities still determined their own curricula, but governments determined the qualification and training which would precede registration. In brief, the emergence of the medical profession, and the state's expanded view of its social responsibilities, neatly complemented each other.

By the time New Guinea was annexed to the German empire and Papua to the British, in 1884, the earlier laissez-faire attitude towards health had substantially passed away. From the outset, the colonial administration would treat public health as a central element of its functions.[5] Many of the shifts described above are exemplified in the career of the first long-term Administrator of British New Guinea (or Papua, to use the later and clearer term). William MacGregor was born the son of a Scots farm labourer, in obscure poverty.[6] Through his native intelligence and the respect of the Scots for scholarship, he was able to study medicine and graduated from Edinburgh University. A reliable income was best provided by the Colonial Service, and MacGregor served as Medical Officer in the Seychelles before he joined Sir Arthur Gordon's fledgling administration of Fiji. His service was eventful, and included public disputes with other doctors in the best nineteenth century style. In Fiji he gained experience in general administration, to supplement his medical expertise. In 1888 therefore he was promoted to Port Moresby, where he was Administrator until 1898, before climbing further through the ranks of colonial administration to crown his career as Governor of Queensland. A Scots background, lowly social origins, and public combativeness were not at all exceptional. Only slightly exceptional was the use of medicine as a spring-board from a labourer's cottage to a Government House, a career which somewhat exaggerates the rise of the medical profession in public esteem.

If the evolution of medical science placed new opportunities in the hands of governments, the particular interests of governments also shaped the direction and focus of medical research and practice. The acquisition of formal colonies in tropical regions (in Africa as well as the Pacific) confronted the new imperialism with large problems. An early colonial doctor in Papua put the problem this way:

> Throughout Australasia the climate of New Guinea is regarded with terror, and the country has much the same reputation, in the antipodes, as the West Coast of Africa formerly enjoyed among ourselves . . . I believe that a certain confusion exists in the popular mind owing to the similarity of names between New Guinea and the Guinea coast of Africa; and the disastrous results which have followed when the discovery of a new gold-field has caused a sudden influx of miners, ignorant and careless in matters of tropical sanitation, have only tended to confirm this unfavourable impression.[7]

How was colonial administration and the exploitation of tropical resources to be accomplished in the face of high mortality rates of Europeans?

A glimmer of hope appeared when Robert Ross demonstrated the role of the anopheles mosquito in the malaria cycle, and when Patrick Manson incriminated the mosquito in the transmission of filariasis.[8] These discoveries came to the attention of the orchestrator of Britain's new imperialism in the 1890s, Joseph Chamberlaim, Her Majesty's Secretary of State for Colonies. By the end of the century, there was an Institute of Tropical Medicine in London, directed by Manson, conducting laboratory research, promoting learned journals, and offering courses in tropical medicine to doctors about to take up positions in the tropics. It will be argued that this was the origin of the worst disaster to befall Melanesians, so the leading features of the new discipline may be worth a moment's reflection.

Robert Ross deduced from his own research, that the way was now open to a general relief of human suffering. Control over water, to prevent stagnant pools from forming, or to move people away from pools which could not be drained, would contribute to the sum of human health: therefore the first priority of tropical administrators must be water control. In practice, colonial administrations paid little attention to public works of this kind, and gave greater status to medical officers than to engineers. Again, the scientific discoveries about mosquito behaviour might have led to intense field-work: in practice they gave rise to laboratory-based experiments, more likely to seek out cures than to prevent infection.

The most serious fault of the new strategy was its disregard for European history. The condition of West Africa, and of New Guinea, which most alarmed Europeans, was substantially that of southern Europe a century earlier: uncontrolled water, untreated sewage, and the diseases of poverty. The tropics dismayed nineteenth-century Europeans, because conditions which had once been universal had now been restricted and seemed strange. The control of water, sewage and food, and the general increase in living standards in western Europe, had not only transformed European lives, but had modified European perceptions. Isolated from an accurate historical model of public health, researchers resorted to the racial explanations which came so naturally to the late Victorians. The research itself was soundly conducted, but the scientific results were cast in the form of contrasts between different racial categories, their predisposition to particular kinds of infection, their varying resistance to it, and their different mortality and morbidity rates. While this research can be illuminating (and much useful research was actually conducted) it turned its back on the social conditions within which hereditary factors operated. As Worboys points out, the structure of research was implicitly racist.[9]

Tropical medical research along these new lines produced some unhappy consequences in colonial Africa. MacGregor spent four years as Governor of Lagos on the West African coast, and his reading of Ross's work on malaria led him to propose extensive swamp drainage. This eminently sensible proposal was countermanded by the Colonial Office, alarmed by the likely expense and more interested in protecting the expatriate enclave than in improving the health of the whole population.[10] Very generally, colonial policy in Africa concentrated on protecting segregated enclaves of expatriates instead of seeking a general increase in health status through public works.[11] And in the settler societies of southern Africa, doctors played a leading role in justifying the segregation of urban communities along racial lines in the first years of this century.[12]

Tropical medicine may have lacked a scientific basis, but it did not lack patronage. The first medical research centre in Australia was founded in Townsville in North Queensland, in 1911: the Australian Institute of Tropical Medicine, created by private capital, popular sentiment, and government subsidy.[13] In Australia, the implicit racism of the discipline was exaggerated by local anxieties, since only in northern Australia was it an open question whether a predominantly white population could establish itself in a tropical environment.[14] It was this question which Dr Anton Breinl and his colleagues and successors addressed in Townsville.

The social tendency of this research was suggested by Breinl's successor, Sir Raphael Cilento, when he summed up the reasons for the successful settlement of North Queensland by people of European descent:

> the absence of any teeming native coloured population, riddled by endemic disease [combined with effective quarantine measures, improved standards of living, and an increase in the Queensland-born population] . . . it was with the arrival of swarms of coloured labourers that the situation became critical.[15]

That perception tied tropical *disease* to tropical *people*. The infections could be prevented if their carriers were physically excluded. During the 1920s the institute became the leading training centre for doctors proceeding to the Australian tropics. Cilento advertised the institute's purpose in these terms:

> From the earliest days of colonisation European diseases were introduced in quantity among the early settlers; various tropical diseases were introduced by the Kanakas from the islands of the Pacific; and by the hordes of Chinese and other Asiatics that poured in before the days of Federation ... Three sets of disease conditions consequently present themselves for control:
>
> (1) those introduced from European countries;
> (2) those introduced from neighbouring tropical lands;
> (3) those indigenous to the country.[16]

The racist language of this scientific analysis obscures the social and environmental conditions which gave rise to most of the infections of the region. The linking of particular 'sets' of disease to particular ethnic communities, perfectly justified the policies of quarantine and segregation.

This perception involved a drastic shift in approach, and in the remedies considered appropriate to tropical medical administration. Once again the shift can be illustrated in the career of William MacGregor a generation earlier. Despite his elevation to a colonial governorship, Mac-Gregor maintained an interest in medical research, and corresponded with his friend Robert Ross, who kept him up to date with scientific developments.[17] At the end of his term in Papua, he was still in good standing with the pioneers of tropical medicine and was invited to address the student body of the new School of Tropical Medicine in London. Most of what he said, however, struck at the assumptions of the new discipline. As against the laboratory methods of tropical medicine, he urged:

> Let me impress upon you the extreme desirableness of becoming experts in the examination of water. Nothing is of greater importance in the tropics ... the quality of the water used by a community may have as much, or nearly as much, influence on them as has the quality of the food they eat or of the air they breathe.

The new discipline was already fascinated by diseases which were thought to be tropical in provenance. As against that perspective, he argued:

> dysentery causes more deaths than any other disease in tropical countries. No other malady is so universally distributed and of such constant occurrence ... [Dysentery has become] the chief agent in the rapid depopulation of the Pacific ... The man who will work out an effective and practical means of dealing with contagious dysentery will be the greatest benefactor of the races that live in the tropics. He may claim to be the saviour of the Pacific Islander, the most lovable man of men now living.

The audience of doctors may have approved his implication that tropical medicine was purely a men's affair but they certainly did not share his focus on indigenous health as the object of administrative effort. The only point on which MacGregor's view coincided with the emerging orthodoxy was the importance of quarantine. He conceded that British authorities always (and properly) opposed the imposition of quarantine, but the tropical dependencies lacked the ample hospital accommodation and the trained officers required to isolate individuals, to disinfect vessels routinely, and in some cases to disinfect whole cargoes. At no point in the published account of his address did MacGregor oppose the evolution of tropical medicine; nor did he explicitly attack its assumptions and procedures; but his exposition of the real problems and opportunities confronting doctors in tropical colonies cut right across the habits of thought which would dominate tropical medicine for half a century.[18]

MacGregor described Chamberlain's purpose as 'curtailing the death-roll of our fellow-citizens in those insalubrious over-sea territories of the empire'. A similar concern animated the German authorities, on whose behalf the great researcher Robert Koch toured the German overseas empire in the first years of this century. It was he who brought the good news of anopheles mosquitoes and of quinine as a prophylactic to German New Guinea.[19] He was not concerned about the endemic malaria which infested Melanesians, but the malaria epidemics which struck down his compatriots. A few years later, when Dr Fleming Jones described medical conditions in Papua (now under Australian rule), he placed Papuans firmly in the category of environmental circumstances which jeopardised the health of Europeans.[20] Dr Anton Breinl, touring the Papuan province of his sphere of influence as Director of the Australian Institute of Tropical Medicine, encouraged a shift of research towards bowel parasites; and his re-direction encouraged further work on bowel parasites among plantation labourers.[21] Yet these scientific developments skirted those general questions of public health which (in the 1980s) we might expect to be paramount.

Combining the roles of Administrator and doctor, MacGregor was a medical strategist without an army. It is not simply the accident of history which made him the last medical strategist for a generation. Fundamentally, the emergence of 'tropical medicine' as a distinct discipline transformed doctors into the decisive agents of colonial policy (whereas engineers, hydrologists, or even nurses might conceivably have exercised that authority); and it transformed doctors from strategists into technicians. A government doctor in a tropical dependency could spend his time and energy on research into the mis-named tropical diseases, sheltered from the knowledge that most of his work was of only marginal significance to the bulk of the population. MacGregor was not the last medical officer who was personally humane and professionally competent, but he was the last for a long time, whose humanity and competence were not blinkered by delight in the technical solution of narrowly defined problems.

With the establishment of colonial administrations, New Guinea and Papua were brought within the scope of imperial medical knowledge, so that their medical officers routinely received circulars from London, regarding the treatment of leprosy, cancer, hookwork, and (by the 1920s) malnutrition.[22] By the 1920s also, there were Pacific regional conferences of medical officers.[23] The chief concern of these conferences was quarantine, and the building of an unbroken quarantine chain. Raphael Cilento observed in 1929, however, that most of the research and international concern had addressed the issue of excluding tropical diseases from Australia: rather little was known about the pattern of infection within the tropical dependencies of the Pacific.[24] Indicative of the prevailing concerns of those in power was the existence in Sydney of the Racial Hygiene Association of New South Wales. As late as the 1930s, this voluntary association flew the names of eminent doctors and public figures at its mast-head, although by that time its chief concern had become birth control (especially for the poor), and the Director of the School of Tropical Medicine seldom attended its functions.[25]

When he was proclaiming the virtues of the discipline which inspired the tropical medical facility in London, Manson asserted (confidently and perhaps correctly) that

> I now believe in the possibility of tropical colonisation by the white race. Heat and moisture are not in themselves the direct cause of any tropical disease. The direct causes of 99% of these diseases are germs . . . To kill them is simply a matter of knowledge and the application of this knowledge.[26]

If we ask why so little of that knowledge was actually applied, part of the answer is the diversion of medical practitioners and planners away from the real causes of infection, towards the study of diseases falsely defined as tropical. MacGregor knew what his contemporaries were forgetting and what his successors neglected – the real basis of Europe's impressive health status. In place of those universally valid measures (which would certainly have proved costly), they adopted a strategy of international quarantine and domestic racial segregation (which was certainly cheaper, and was perfectly in tune with the racist notions of the day).[27] It is not so much the programmes which tropical medicine validated, as the opportunities which it excluded, which condemned Melanesians to persistent ill-health while the health of Australians improved dramatically. Maoris were the only South Pacific population which was not subjected to 'tropical medicine'. The rapid improvement of their health, nutrition and numbers from about 1900 onwards suggests the benefits to be gained through 'temperate' public health measures, and the grievous social cost of 'tropical medicine'.[28] The following chapters will suggest what price was paid by two generations of Papua New Guineans.

3
Early colonial medical administration

Before colonial administration was attempted, it was already clear that Europeans and their servants would suffer acutely from malaria, and in some circumstances from dysentery. The first resident European, the Russian scientist (and disciple of Tolstoy), Nikolai Nikolayevich Miklouho-Maclay, was conveyed to the north coast in 1871, with two man-servants. The Polynesian soon died, and the surviving Swede fell chronically ill. Maclay's health was seriously undermined, and he concluded that

> It is not the Papuans or the tropical heat or the impassable forests that guard the coasts of New Guinea. Their mighty ally protecting them from foreign invaders is the pale cold, first shivering and then burning fever.[1]

Within a few months, the Polynesian pastors and teachers established on the coast of the Papuan Gulf by the London Missionary Society, had to endure devastating mortality rates from malaria. They were familiar with mosquitoes – perhaps too familiar – but not with anopheles, and took quite inadequate precautions.[2] And from the late 1870s there was a series of gold rushes from northern Australia. The prospectors were casual and hasty in arranging sanitation, and fell like nine-pins to dysentery.[3] One vivid account (from a slightly later date, 1889) describes the complete collapse of a whole mining community. John Cameron, a young Victorian adventurer, held minor office on one of the islands in Milne Bay:

> Our island of Sudest is nearly worked out. We have only 180 men on the field at present, and a hundred of those are down with fever and dysentery. I held two inquests this week: one man shot himself while delirious with fever, the other died of general debility.[4]

Colonial administrations were born in crises of fever, which largely explains the defensive, self-interested style of the first health measures. Advice from other tropical colonies reinforced the fear, and pointed towards the possible remedies.[5]

German New Guinea was administered as a commercial venture, by the New Guinea Company, which envisaged a plantation colony resembling Java in the Dutch East Indies. Until the 1890s, it was commonly believed by Europeans that malaria was caused by 'miasma' in the air, best avoided by living at high altitudes, or at least in raised houses.[6] That perception did not encourage suitable precautions, and the settlers paid a doleful price. By July 1887, every European at Constantinhafen was fevered. At Finschhafen four years later, 13 of the 45 Europeans died of malaria in a period of three months, and the survivors fled. Dr Schellong concluded 'Malaria has conquered!'[7] Among the victims was the only doctor in the settlement. Administrator von Schleinitz had already been forced into retirement by broken health. The little colony simply could not sustain losses on this scale, quite apart from the high mortality rates among indentured labourers. The corner was turned soon after the visit by Dr Robert Koch in 1899–1900. He and his colleague Dr Dempwolff brought news of Robert Ross's discoveries, and imposed a regime of regular quinine prophylaxis.[8]

Even then the settlers could survive only at the cost of sharp discomfort. Quinine could be ingested as a bitter liquid, or in tablet form – but the tablet was often useless, passing straight through to the bed pan.[9] They suspected that the bitter medicine might provoke blackwater fever, while warding off malaria. Those who persisted with quinine (and not everybody could stomach it) sometimes suffered severe side-effects – ringing or roaring in the ears, deafness, dizziness, disturbed vision, headache, nausea, diarrhoea or skin rashes. They submitted to the medication only because an infected population was even worse off – bloodless, breathless, listless, often nursing enlarged spleens, but otherwise terribly emaciated.[10]

A plantation economy would depend upon a large labour force, which the company recruited in Singapore and the Dutch East Indies. The company had to provide for the health of these labourers. Medical staff were recruited

> in the financial interests of the Company, which are better served by keeping the labourers in good health than by saving a doctor's salary. The Board of Directors therefore engaged a second doctor [in 1888] and after his departure they had to consider appointing a replacement.[11]

The morbidity and mortality rates among these imported labourers were dangerously high (although their precise levels are a matter of dispute).[12] Illness was not simply a consequence of New Guinean conditions, since 'labour is not always selected in Singapore with the necessary care, so that repeatedly shipments have contained a majority of people weakened by age or illness and unfit for work'.[13] Linked by direct shipping services with Java and Singapore, German New Guinea was peculiarly vulnerable to imported infection. In the early 1890s smallpox entered the territory: 'The disease first attacked the Melanesians with great severity and then spread in waves, first to [Bogadjim, near Madang] then extending to the native villages.' Lymph was brought from Java, and a mass vaccination campaign was launched, as far as the government's writ ran.[14] Until the twentieth century, however, the government's writ did not run very far, nor very fast, beyond the harbour enclaves. Quarantine became the most common and effective strategy of medical officers. That strategy was certainly more important than the few, small (and racially segregated) hospitals, at the leading centres of administration. It was quinine and quarantine which permitted German New Guinea first to survive and then – on the islands, if not on the mainland – to flourish in the first years of this century.[15]

German annexation of New Guinea spurred the Australian colonists to lever a reluctant British government into the protectorate of British New Guinea in 1884. Port Moresby was selected as the centre of administration, because of its 'comparative healthiness' and easy access to Cooktown in northern Queensland. In the event, the climate proved enervating: the first annual report prayed for sugar plantations as a device for driving out fever. The first budget provided nearly £250 for medical attendants and almost £100 for medical stores. In a total budget of £15,000, this was ludicrously inadequate. As if to prove the point, the first Commissioner died before he could write a report.[16]

Papuan administration was chronically starved of funds, and medical provisions were as rudimentary as everything else. After the departure of MacGregor in 1898, morale was depressed by the suicide of an acting Administrator, by Britain's manifest lack of interest, and by federal Australia's tardiness in accepting its responsibilities. The budget eventually provided for a doctor, and from 1900 onwards a doctor's name would appear briefly on the establishment, until the new man found something better elsewhere.[17] A cadre of committed doctors accrued only slowly. Walter Mersh Strong, a graduate of Cambridge and St Thomas's Hospital, sometime assistant in the Skin and Electrical Department of St Thomas's, arrived on an ethnographic expedition in 1904. He found this remote outpost congenial, and was employed as an Assistant Resident Magistrate. He reverted to medicine in 1910, took a diploma in Tropical Medicine and Hygiene in London in 1914, and rose to the heights of Chief Medical Officer for Papua. In that administration, since everyone was expected to perform several functions, he relished the opportunity to blend the work of Chief Medical Officer, Chief Quarantine Officer, and Government Anthropologist. He retired in the territory, and died there, senile, after the Pacific War.[18]

A similar drifter who put down roots in Papua was Ralph Bellamy. He turned up in 1905, having abandoned medical studies and gold prospecting. Engaged as an Assistant Resident Magistrate for the Trobriand Islands, he practised as a medical officer and served until 1938, with interruptions to fight in the Great War and to complete his medical degree and a Townsville Diploma in Tropical Medicine.[19] There was also a Mr J. Taafe, thought to have been a medical student, who practised medicine on Woodlark Island (Murua) from 1902 until he died in 1921.[20] By 1913 Dr Eric Giblin had also arrived in Samarai (the commercial centre of early colonial Papua), to begin forty years of medical service to the country.[21] Other doctors came and went. Their calibre may be inferred from Dr Sam Lambert's description immediately after the Great War:

The whole medical service was pared down to an excellent Chief Medical Officer with nothing to work with, a Judgment Day prophet in charge of the local hospital, and one physician for each of three far-flung districts. These five, with a couple of nurses and two European dispensers, were supposed to service the 90,000 odd square miles. The officer at Samarai was efficiently modern: the other three were elderly hacks. This was typical of the general situation over the South Pacific.[22]

As in Australia, so in Papua: hospitals were built wherever the expatriate population could subscribe funds – Samarai, Murua (during the gold rush), and Port Moresby. As late as 1920, the two surviving European hospitals each had an average in-patient population of two.[23] That may have been as many as the staff could cope with. Governor Murray later remembered having to ban Dr Mathews (the 'Judgment Day prophet' of Lambert's account) from Port Moresby hospital.[24] Papuan patients did not seek to be hospitalised, nor could they afford to pay medical fees; so the government built small native hospitals close to the European hospitals at Samarai and Port Moresby.

We have considered doctors and hospitals. In point of fact, the cutting edge of European medicine in this era was neither the doctor nor the hospital, but the trained nurse. In the days before the modern miracle drugs, sick people were not doctored and drugged back to good health, but nursed. It was the paucity of nurses, rather than the shortage of physicians, which most severely hampered the colonial administration. Only the missions could lure trained female nurses to the territories. In Papua, Anglican nurses stemmed one of the worst outbreaks of dysentery on one of the gold fields;[25] but government nurses, when they were employed at all, were confined to European hospitals. The same difficulty afflicted German New Guinea. In 1889 a mission offered two nursing sisters to the company 'on condition that their personal safety there is guaranteed by the presence of European women'. This meant, in effect, that the nurses would only tend white patients. The role of the nurses is implied by the company's delight that 'the active presence of female nurses would also remove or reduce many inadequacies in the hospital arising from unsatisfactory management of the kitchen and laundry'.[26] Not surprisingly, nurses did not stay long. In desperation, the German authorities began training 'medical *tultuls*' in the villages under their control. Their functions were mainly first aid, and the swift reporting of untoward infection.[27] They were no substitute for trained nurses. The absence of nurses also ensured that the government services would make no provision whatever for maternal or child health – which was precisely the area of public health which was being transformed in Australia and New Zealand during the first half of the twentieth century.[28]

Equally, infection rates might have been reduced by an energetic programme of public works, draining swamps and regulating water and sewage. That strategy was implicit in Robert Ross's view of malaria control, but was superseded by a (cheaper) strategy of urban segregation in British tropical colonies.[29] In both New Guinea and Papua, government budgets were far too small to permit a programme of preventative public works.[30] By default, therefore, public health remained the province of doctors rather than engineers.

Medical authorities were kept very busy during the first generation of colonialism, in crisis-management. When there was no urgent crisis to ride, doctors devoted themselves to a scatter of research: bowel parasites interested Strong, while Bellamy tackled the severe problem of venereal diseases on the Trobriand Islands.[31] Otherwise they educated settlers in the use of quinine, established quarantine procedures, and simply advised Europeans to live at least a quarter of a mile away from Melanesians.[32]

The fragile nature of this holding operation was revealed when the Great War broke out, and a large detachment of Australian soldiers occupied German New Guinea. The small German police detachments offered little resistance:

> the native troops were demoralised, and ... to keep them together as a military unit required the unceasing vigilance of the white soldiers, among whom many were disabled by dysentery and malaria.[33]

In the largest skirmish before the German capitulation at Rabaul, the only Australian battle casualty was suffered: Dr Pockley was killed after he had lent his Red Cross insignia to a wounded colleague.[34] The men of the Australian Naval and Military Expeditionary Force began to suffer only after they had achieved their military objective. Happily, the invasion force arrived in the dry season, and was withdrawn before the rains, so they had few opportunities to fall sick.[35] It was the relieving detachment – Tropical Force, of about 600 – which had the worst experience. By January 1915, 60 per cent of them were laid low by malaria, and although the epidemic was brought under control at Rabaul, problems persisted in Madang, and especially at Angoram, where the small garrison had to be withdrawn after two deaths from malaria.[36] Malaria was followed by amoebic dysentery, probably introduced from the Middle East by troops invalided out of that theatre.[37] Quaintly, a ship carrying reinforcements had to be quarantined in Rabaul harbour, until a measles epidemic ran its course on board.[38] By the end of the war, however, strict military discipline and forced labour to fill swamps and collect rubbish around garrison posts had brought both malaria and dysentery under control. It was plausible for Colonel MacKenzie to conclude that

> Never again, in a fight against the attacks of a treacherous tropical climate, in relation both to its own personnel and to the native population ... will an Australian administration be handicapped to the same extent as was the military administration.[39]

We suggested that the chief element in maintaining relatively good health among Melanesians was their isolation. Given the enthusiasm of the new colonial authorities for quarantine and segregation, we might imagine that Melanesian well-being was secure. In reality, quarantine was successful in isolating Australia from Melanesian infections, but was less effective in the other direction. We have seen that smallpox found its way to German New Guinea in the 1890s. It has also been suggested that either smallpox or possibly chickenpox touched the south coast of Papua shortly before colonial administration.[40] With greater confidence we can point to dysentery as the most dangerous exogenous infection, not only during MacGregor's period in the 1890s, but right through to the Great War, promoted especially by chaotic sanitary conditions on the gold-fields.[41]

Although there were few systematic attempts at a population census, early colonial authorities often formed the impression that depopulation was occurring, occasionally on an alarming scale. Governor Hahl in German New Guinea, for instance, stated the problem in the bleakest terms:

> The country exhibits an abundance of fertile soil with high rainfall and a good supply of water. But the population is sparse, of inferior quality, and diminishing.[42]

Hahl made the connection between depopulation and venereal disease. That diagnosis led him to prohibit the recruitment of women (other than the wives of male labourers) for work outside their home villages. That restriction – implicitly an attack on concubinage – was more oppressive than the planters would tolerate.

In Papua, special hospitals catered for venereal diseases. The nature of these hospitals is revealed by the use of Port Moresby gaol hospital when other isolation wards were unavailable.

> Some few of the venereal patients come in voluntarily but most of the cases are discovered by magistrates while on patrol work and as their detection is associated, in the native mind, with crime and its punishment, there is no doubt that many cases are concealed. The special hospitals [at Samarai, and in the Trobriand Islands] are keeping venereal diseases [sic] in check, to some extent, but it is not being eradicated and is not likely to be, especially as it is being continually reintroduced.[43]

But as Bellamy got the Trobriands health-care system into operation, treatment became less punitive and more therapeutic.[44]

One of the most serious diseases introduced in these early colonial days was tuberculosis.[45] Papua New Guinea was one of very few places on earth, where the 'white death' was not endemic in the early twentieth century. Expatriates inevitably brought it with them, providing multiple foci for infection; and Polynesian teachers and pastors were among the most thoroughly infected of the immigrants. Just as dysentery flourished in the new social and economic structures (the mining camps and plantations), so tuberculosis enjoyed the opportunities presented by colonial social organisation. In one village, it was observed that a victim was effectively quarantined by his peers; but the plantation barracks, the school rooms of the teachers, and even the convent of an order of nuns, assisted the rapid dissemination of the bacillus. The connections between colonialism and tuberculosis became abundantly clear in the 1930s, through the work of two capable epidemiologists. They were delighted to discover that the disease was virtually absent from the highlands, only recently explored , and they found that Hanuabada (by this time a series of Christian, urban villages abutting Port Moresby) was the most heavily infected part of the dependency.[46]

The progress of diseases through the country was erratic, depending largely on existing linkages between village communities. Dr Clement visited Goilala in 1935. He was about fifty miles out of Port Moresby when he noticed that yaws

> had made but little progress inland; altitude may explain this, but more probably it is the absence of that intimate contact between peoples of the mountain districts and the coast so necessary for the spread of the disease . . . At the next village along the road, several cases of framboesia were encountered – all in natives who had recently attended a dance visited by coastal natives.[47]

From this region, links to the south were irregular. More frequent contact was maintained with people on the northern slopes of the mountains, and some cases of poliomyelitis could be traced along this route. The implication of this pattern is that non-colonial transmission routes were often too sporadic to ensure the spread of available infections to all susceptible populations, especially those forms of infection which required frequent or sustained physical contact. However, new routes could sometimes carry heavy traffic. During the 1920s Dr Cilento investigated the health of people on a cluster of tiny islands west of Manus in the Bismarck Archipelago. They had experienced little colonial contact, but even irregular interaction had permitted malaria and venereal disease to bring the island communities to the verge of extinction.[48]

That episode should warn us not to define the issue too precisely as one between endemic and exogenous disease. Colonialism did not simply permit the introduction of entirely new diseases (tuberculosis, smallpox, measles and others) but also allowed the more even redistribution of endemic infections into enclaves which had hitherto been isolated.[49] The mechanism for the introduction, dissemination, and redistribution of infection was the mobilisation of labour for mining, for plantation work, and for general employment by the colonists and their government. And that mechanism was much more effective than the frantic attempts of the health authorities to stamp out epidemics once they occurred. It was extremely fortunate that so few colonial officers, missionaries, or coastal employees found their way into the highlands before the 1930s, for they would certainly have created more ill-health than they could cure. On balance, the medical institutions in the early days of colonialism were rather like band-aids. The impressive feats of public health which were transforming the lives of Europeans and of white Australians were simply not attempted in Melanesia. Medical institutions simply attempted to limit the destructive consequences which would necessarily follow from new forms of social organisation and social interaction. Colonialism itself was a health hazard, which colonial medical services were ill-equipped to suppress.

4
The political economy of health in Papua between the wars

The search for the mainspring of medical policies and programmes must begin with the colonial state, which employed most of the doctors who declared the policies and launched the programmes, and which influenced the behaviour of mission doctors and nurses. It is necessary, therefore, to describe the general purpose of the colonial state and its financial basis. This approach assumes that the colonial state directs its resources (including medical skills) towards the needs of the fledgling colonial economy. When we test that assumption, however, it proves unsatisfactory: it is impossible to construe medical programmes *simply* and mechanically as the state's contribution to capitalism. We adopt that approach to see how far it will take us, and to gauge the extent of doctors' autonomy in policymaking. Since there were two colonial states from 1884 until the Pacific War in the 1940s, we also take the opportunity to consider each on its own in order to seek out comparisons and contrasts. What follows, therefore, is an investigation of the 'political economy' of health policies and programmes setting matters of public health in the constitutional and economic circumstances of each of the dependencies.

British New Guinea, the south-eastern quarter of New Guinea, was a Cinderella among British dependencies. From 1884 when it became a protectorate, this 'oddity of empire' was administered by British officers, and paid for (grudgingly) by the Australian colonies. The new Commonwealth government accepted responsibility for Papua in 1906.[1] Neither that government nor private business had surplus capital to export to Papua. Few Australians would brave an unhealthy environment, where gold was unreliable and the land was not freehold. Alluvial gold supported the export economy until the Great War; small-scale plantation production became its frail backbone between the wars. Even including a small annual grant from the Commonwealth, total revenue was small: expenditure shrank from £158,964 in 1927–28, to £121,198 during the worst of the Depression in 1933–34. In the last full year before the Second World War, the budget only just regained the level of the 1920s.[2] Lacking the capital for large-scale plantation development by Australians, Governor Murray steadily shifted towards the encouragement (or coercion) of small-holder production by Papuans.[3] Economic development was so laggard that 'a casual visitor seeing a village . . . in 1910 and returning again in 1940 would have noticed few changes.'[4] The islands and coastal strips were regularly administered; most of the interior was occasionally explored.

Medical services enjoyed a generous proportion of the frugal budget; but even 11 per cent of the 1933–34 budget yielded only £13,758.[5] Like every other aspect of colonial rule, medical work was affected by Murray's preference for ambidextrous officers who could perform at least two jobs adequately, rather than one job well. Walter Mersh Strong, Chief Medical Officer for most of the years of peace, doubled as Government Anthropologist. Robert Black points out (with cruel precision) that this would have been an excellent combination, had Strong possessed more than a smattering of either discipline.[6] The first casualty of amateurism was research. Between Breinl's visit in 1913, and Clements' in 1935, the research records consisted entirely of part-time work by Strong (on helminth parasites in faeces), and Bellamy (on venereal disease and demography in the Trobriand islands).[7] Strong was very much Murray's kind of man, not so much a specialist as a man of wide-ranging curiosity. When Murray fell ill in 1913, he wrote in a letter that 'Strong says that I had a complaint called Alastrim or Kaffir Milk Pox – a little known disease which he found described in a recent book on tropical medicine'.[8] The patient was a champion boxer who lived on until he was 80, so the diagnosis did not need to be very accurate, so long as the prescription was moderate.

The distribution of resources can be seen in the analysis of medical expenditure in selected years in table 1.[9] Hospital duties tied down much of the department, rather inefficiently. Even after Woodlark hospital closed (in the 1920s, when the gold was exhausted), the department had to maintain two hospitals in Samarai and another two in Port Moresby. By the end of the Strong era, Port Moresby European hospital had an average of 2 in-patients at a time, Port Moresby Native hospital had 61; while Samarai European catered to 2.6 patients, and Samarai Native to 123.[10] Strong could not evade these responsibilities, but he allowed hospitals lower priority than extension work. He stopped tending to hospital patients himself, leaving the single medical officer in Port Moresby to cope with hospital work and private practice.[11] European hospitals were cut more severely than other elements of the medical programme, to cope with the Depression.

There were never more than five doctors in the territory, and often fewer. A gold mine was developed on the remote island of Misima in Milne Bay during the 1930s, so a doctor had to be posted there. Following a dispute with the mining company, Dr Alec May's duties were spelt out for him. He was obliged to supervise the native hospital, treat Papuans in the government hospital, examine all labourers prior to indenture, conduct post-mortems as required by the coroner, perform the duties of Health Officer for the island, perform (free of charge) any work required by the Administration, inspect the mines ('probably once a month'), inspect the barracks of the mining property, inspect prisoners and Crown servants and their quarters once a month, report on any Papuan on government premises

Table 1

| | 1928–29 | 1933–34 |
	£	£
Medical and sanitary staff	4,907	4,722
European hospitals	3,069	1,956
Native hospitals	2,922	2,395
Travelling staff	7,277	4,686
Total medical expenditure	18,175	13,759
Total government expenditure	152,949	121,198

(and give evidence in court, if necessary), be the private practitioner for everyone on the island, and – if a European hospital were built – supervise it.[12] These were exceptionally wide duties, yet doctors in Papua were paid less than their counterparts in New Guinea. It is scarcely surprising that so few remained in Papua, or that some served less than adequately.[13] Since hospitals existed, they had to be staffed, either by Australian female nurses (in European hospitals only) or by partly-trained Papuan orderlies. The other personnel consisted largely of that distinctive category, the European medical assistant. These men might be medical students who had abandoned their studies, or ex-servicemen who had been ward orderlies, or artisans who had taken a St John's Ambulance certificate. Most had to be bachelors.[14] A medical assistant might deputise for a doctor in his absence: the distinction between a fully qualified practitioner and an assistant was not sharp. More commonly, the medical assistant was an extension officer, leading patrols into the hinterland of the little towns on the coast.

The establishment increased significantly during the 1930s, when Strong organised the training of a cadre of Papuan medical assistants – about 50 by 1936 – to supplement the more expensive Australians. Colonial circumstances ensured that the Papuan medical assistants received only the bare minimum of training – perhaps 12 months' instruction after primary schooling.[15] (There was no high school in Papua; settler opinion was hostile to the students visiting Australia at all.) Strong made the widest possible use of them: as early as 1926, three Papuans led their own five-month patrol, meticulously recording their procedures; and one accompanied Strong to address a medical congress in Australia. For the most part they performed rural extension work, and a few made up prescriptions under supervision.[16]

Given these constraints, medical administration relied heavily upon the voluntary participation of the community. Sensibly, the Department prepared a *Handbook on the treatment and prevention of disease in Papua when medical advice is unobtainable* (Port Moresby, 1917). For Papuans, printed advice was irrelevant. Few Papuans could read the advice of the first *Papuan Villager* (15 February 1929) that

The people must not fight with spears and arrows any more; they must not pretend to kill one another with bad magic; they must not bury the dead inside the village. These are bad fashions.

Strong commented that:

You can take a horse to water, but you cannot make him drink ... the Government pays me to look after [Papuans'] health and I am quite willing to help them all I can, but if they will not come for treatment it is their own concern, and as far as I am concerned it merely saves trouble.[17]

It requires an imaginative leap to return to the limited treatments available to Strong and his colleagues in the 1930s. The *Handbook* listed 29 drugs and mixtures, and 18 kinds of dressing and salve. What bleeding was for nineteenth century practitioners, purging was in the early twentieth. Purging was recommended in the case of fever, in the event of dysentery, and even (a peculiarly unpleasant one) for the widespread colonial disease, Malingering. The few medicaments which had no purgative effect, were to be taken with a purge: this was the era of Epsom Salts.[18] Strong was not unusual in this enthusiasm, and he was well-regarded by Lambert,[19] and by those who survived his heroic prescriptions.

The main thrust of medical strategy was quarantine and segregation, the physical separation of potential and actual foci of infection. The received wisdom was that Europeans could survive tropical environments, if only they were isolated from tropical people.[20] Accordingly, Strong advised settlers to keep their distance from Papuans if they valued their health. There was also a lively fear, at least until the 1930s, that Papuans might be dying out in the face of introduced disease.[21] Since very few infections could actually be cured, segregation seemed the only practicable strategy: it involved residential segregation by race, strict control over shipping, and the building of quarantine facilities (on the Trobriand islands, at Gesila in Milne Bay, and on Gemo island near Port Moresby).[22]

Throughout the 1920s, Papuan medical strategy and programmes were decisively influenced by the Rockefeller Foundation, which was conducting a crusade against hookworm infestation across the world.[23] It followed a very successful programme in north Queensland, promoting the construction and use of pit-latrines. Not for the last time, a scientific programme was extended from sparsely-settled Australia (where it was effective) to the densely inhabited Pacific islands (where it was not). Oil of chemopodium was administered to plantation labourers, and to the residents of villages within range of the patrols. Evangelists in the crusade lectured workers and villagers on hookworm and personal sanitation, and encouraged the use of pit latrines. Since the patrols were irregular, they achieved the temporary relief of many Papuan men, but failed to eradicate hookworm, as Lambert eventually conceded.[24]

However limited its success, the hookworm campaign expressed the intention of the Government to encourage the plantation industry. Strong was careful to assemble up-to-date information about diet, noting advances in the treatment of beri-beri and the progress of vitamin research generally. This information was disseminated (along with the *Handbook*) to planters and the managers of mines.[25] Since the Department relied on the voluntary cooperation of employers, there was no question of prosecuting managers who permitted unsatisfactory diets. Instead, Strong appealed to their self-interest in a healthy and vigorous labour line. Much the same vision encouraged managers to cooperate enthusiastically in the hookworm campaign.[26]

One of the compelling attractions of the hookworm campaign was that it was technically simple, requiring only a large stock of Epsom Salts to wash down the oil of chemopodium, and a good microscope to count bowel parasites in faeces samples. The other great campaign of these years – yaws – shared that simplicity. By the end of the Great War it was possible to administer a single injection of an arsenical compound, which cleared up yaws as if by magic. During 1922 Dr Harse treated all the children in Poreporena village (near Port Moresby), with spectacular success. 360 children were injected, and the resident missionary reported that every case responded well. The populace responded even better: mothers mobbed the hospital, clamouring to have their children injected; and people came from the whole coastal region to be treated.[27] The acting Administrator recognised that little skill was required for giving the injections, so he proposed that mission personnel be involved, in villages inaccessible to the medical people.[28] Again the response was dramatic. Strong reported the effectiveness of the new compound M&B 914, much cheaper than arsenicals and almost as successful. 1,568 patients each received a single injection, 87 per cent were cured, 16 per cent improved, while 3 per cent experienced no change. Two hundred people received a second dose, which cured or improved the condition in 95 per cent of cases.[29] The social response was equally gratifying. As news of the injection spread, medical patrols were guaranteed an enthusiastic reception, with people lining up for treatment, even in villages which resented every other manifestation of colonial administration.[30] Every previous medical patrol had been perceived as an intrusion: venereal patients would be incarcerated, and faeces samples were collected and removed for some unfathomable magical purpose. Now the needle was seen as an unmixed blessing.

This technical capacity gave a curious slant to medical extension work. The records for 1925–26 present the following statistics:

49,518 hookworm treatments,
12,643 yaws treatments,
186 cases of venereal disease,
51 cases of everything else.[31]

Since the hookworm treatment was often ineffective, and yaws was more commonly an inconvenience than anything more serious, the extension work accomplished little except impressive statistics. To some extent also, medical services were inhibited by the need to gain some tacit support from Papuans. On behalf of the administration, Constance Fairhall of the London Missionary Society (LMS) directed Gemo Island isolation hospital near Port Moresby, in the late 1930s. The general intention was to isolate tuberculosis cases, and this ran counter to the opinion of the villagers affected by the disease:

> Untrue and fear-inspiring stories are still being circulated about Gemo, though one or two of these stories, we admit, originated from our own mistakes, such as the mistake we made when, through sheer force of circumstance, we buried one of our cases at sea. For weeks no fishermen came near the island, and there was much consternation in the local villages . . . through fear of catching Tubercular fish . . . Most of the troubles predicted . . . have not eventuated . . . but the bringing of hordes of young children to see patients has been a nuisance, and is most unwise. [And] at first we tried desperately hard to stick to our principles, and to keep . . . very ill cases, who came to us from the local villages, until death, the bodies then being taken straight back to their own cemetery . . . However, we found that this created a great deal of unhappiness and difficulty, and, therefore, much against our will, we feel that the time is perhaps, not yet, and now we allow very ill cases to be taken home just before the end.[32]

How did Papuans experience medical services? Unless they sought treatment (most probably for yaws), they might not experience the services at all. A young villager in Rigo district, very close to Port Moresby, crippled as an infant, attended the full range of LMS schools, and evaded treatment until he began to train as a teacher, when the mission found him a pair of crutches and referred him to a doctor.[33] If a cripple on a mission station in Rigo could escape medication, then the surveillance system as a whole must have been worse than lax. And there was every incentive to avoid treatment. Strong's medicines were almost all purgatives. Government gaols had diets much better than those which prevailed on plantations,[34] but few enjoyed the experience. Most patients who were removed from their villages (for venereal diseases or leprosy) were detained in isolation hospitals until they died or recovered. Native hospitals were run by slightly trained orderlies, and women in particular were reluctant to place themselves at the mercy of these strangers.[35]

The reputation of the native hospitals can be inferred from admission statistics. Port Moresby Native Hospital in 1918–19 was in no way exceptional in the wider record. According to the *Annual Report* for that year, the following patients were admitted:

Indentured labourers	524 ⎫	=	71%
Time-expired indentured labourers	36 ⎭		
Rejected recruits	57		
Prisoners	44		
Government employees	162	=	20%
'Non-Papuan coloured'	10		
'Villagers'	38	=	5%
	871 patients		

Apart from the 38 'villagers', Papuans entered hospital only because their employers sent them there.

The small department necessarily relied on the support of other agencies (such as the plantations) to function at all. Its most effective and enthusiastic allies were the missionary societies. Providing village-based cooperation, transport networks and accommodation, and the most effective lobbying in the territory, the missions were essential to the operation of a medical strategy of any kind.

Christian missions have often taken literally the injunction to heal the sick; and especially to 'suffer the little children'.[36] The earliest missionaries to Papua had their work cut out to heal themselves. Before 1914, few had any medical preparation for life in Papua. Married missionaries often contrived to send their wives and children to Australia or Europe. That was a wise precaution, as Langmore notes that ten of the first 65 babies born to missionaries in Papua died in their first year of life, and 5 more died in early childhood.[37] Missionaries soon turned to rescuing other people's children, either from interment with their mothers, or from social conditions considered inimical to the Christian life.[38] From the 1890s onwards, missions were almost the sole source of medical assistance apart from the government's work on behalf of a healthy labour line. Those services were, above all, child-centred.[39]

Strong had considered maternal and child health from an ethnographic point of view, very early in his Papuan career. A quarter of a century passed before he considered them as a doctor, possibly because of his bachelor condition, or perhaps because the Cambridge curriculum did not consider this field.[40] His belated judgment was that the high infant mortality rate was the problem. One method was to pay a 'baby bonus' to *fathers* of large families.[41] But the problem could also be tackled by 'teaching the Papuan better ways of feeding, and treating infants and young children'. He reasoned that this work 'could best be done in cooperation with and by the Missions', provided always that no great strain was placed upon the budget. He proposed to appoint one or two nurses at appropriate mission stations, whose work 'should consist mainly in the matter of rearing children'. Relatively little return would be achieved through the work of the white nurses themselves: their important function would be to train Papuan girls. This work could not be done effectively by the government, because the 'ordinary trained nurse has to earn her living and would expect a high salary. Unless of the Missionary type she would hardly be content to settle down for life to work for natives' and in any case the missions were best able to provide rural transport and housing. Almost as an afterthought – but a revealing one – he turned his mind to the actual production of children:

> Perhaps such nurses could help in the matter of teaching the population how to treat the expectant mother, and to improve the native methods of conducting labour. But I would deprecate any attempt to bring such cases into

> Hospitals or to seriously interfere with native methods without carefully counting the cost.[42]

It transpired that the missions had been doing a great deal of work, of which the government was unaware. Early in 1931 Governor Murray was delighted to discover that every Catholic mission station had a nursing sister (including 'some qualified'), who visited villages and tended sick children. During these visits, the sister

> does her best to help expectant mothers: they give them advice. Native women also come and consult the sister about their peculiar troubles. As to conducting labour ... the sister usually is not allowed to, in easy confinements, owing to the adverse native mentality. But, when the confinement is laborious, the nursing sister is called in, and, then, her help well accepted.

Murray's surprise was the greater because, as a Governor, a Catholic and a friend of many of the priests, he had not in a quarter of a century had occasion to ask what the nuns did with their time, or what assistance Papuan women received.[43]

Other missions were also active in matters of child and maternal health. The Seventh Day Adventists, for example, served a coastal population south-east of Port Moresby. Their training programme distinguished between boys (who were taught first aid) and girls (who learned to look after children). That service seems also to have been child-centred, since only 30 maternity cases were recorded in 1933–34, in a total of 12,768 cases; and the report dwelt on infant care, while failing to mention maternity.[44] Too much confidence should not be placed in these records, however, as two-thirds of all treatments were for tinea, and a full quarter were 'miscellaneous'.

Medical care was also well developed at Kwato mission in Milne Bay (an independent LMS station). Within sight of Samarai and its three hospitals, the Abel family built their own hospital. This apparent duplication is explained in part by the Abels' horror of the rough-hewn medical orderlies, who terrorised women patients in the government hospitals. For a while in the 1930s they employed Dr Berkeley Vaughan; but more commonly Kwato hospital was staffed by female trained nurses. The medical purpose was not so much to provide hospital care, as to train female nurses. Commonly, the nurses then married the Papuan managers of mission out-stations, which consisted of a plantation, a church, a school, and a clinic.[45]

The complaint of the Catholics, that village women preferred not to have European assistance in child-birth, seems curious. In other missions, women did intervene in child-birth as well as in child-care. These interventions were mainly informal, often spontaneous, and sustained by very little expertise in midwifery. An arresting example is to be found in the recollections of one woman missionary, from the late 1930s.[46] Mr and Mrs Deasey had received some medical instruction in Australia, in order to medicate themselves in their remote mission station. On arrival in the Gulf, they found alarming child-birth and nurturing practices. Before a woman produced her first child, she received some advice, including advice from men, on what to expect. To hasten the baby's arrival, the mother carried heavy loads in the late stages of pregnancy. At the onset of labour, she took herself to a hut on her husband's land, carrying the standard equipment: ginger, sugar-cane, a sliver of bamboo, string, sago, and a coconut. Near kin followed her, but not too closely. If labour was protracted, her kin would assist by beating her on the back 'to waken the baby'. Otherwise she delivered her baby alone, removed and buried the placenta, and carried the infant home. Mrs Deasey was not allowed to attend a birth, until she managed to break the taboo in the case of the wife of a houseboy. The baby was within the usual range of weight for the community at that time (three to four pounds) and was born in the usual weather conditions (rain). When the baby thrived, despite the presence of a man in the house, a trickle and then a flood of women sought Mrs Deasey's assistance at birthing. The episode embodies a number of common colonial themes: the absence of a midwifery tradition (despite Murray's and Strong's vague references to harmless rituals),[47] procedures likely to entail devastating maternal and child mortality rates, impulsive intervention by a woman with little pertinent training – and a most eager response. Some Papuan traditions were more honoured in the breach...[48]

In judging the Papuan medical service, it has to be conceded that Strong stretched his tiny resources to the utmost, seeking always to expand his services beyond the expatriate enclaves and the labour lines, to the great masses of ordinary villagers. It must also be said that the personnel were enthusiastic amateurs, with the weaknesses as well as the strengths of their amateurism. As late as 1940, the government architect in Port Moresby believed that malaria was produced by impurities in the soil – until the Director General of Health for the Commonwealth brought him up to date with nineteenth century science.[49] An insuperable problem was the absence of either laboratory facilities or competent training centres. One of the few doctors employed by the missions wrote in these terms to the School of Public Health and Tropical Medicine in Sydney, in 1935

> I am sending by the first opportunity a few specimens. Two are early Papuan embryos which I thought you might like for the Museum. Another is a tumour ... There is also a smaller similar tumour ... The last specimen is a penis, and it is cases like this which make it very distressing that we have no laboratory in the whole of this Territory. The case was a middle-aged man with, probably, chronic Gonorrhea and a resultant ulceration of the glans, prepuse etc. But as local treatment of the ulcerated part for about ten days left it still stony hard in one part I felt that it was better to run the risk of an unnecessary mutilation rather than lose the chance of stopping the spread of a possible carcinoma.[50]

Behind these sorry accounts lurks an impersonal culprit: a pointless colonialism.[51] Australian lack of interest in Papua before the Pacific War affects the record at every turn. Responsibility was assumed for a colonial dependency, but no adequate funding was provided. An alien administration was imposed, but without professional competence. A medical department was unleashed, although its personnel lacked expertise. While people died of exogenous disease, the few medical administrators pursued hookworm with a dedication which deserved a better focus. Scragg describes the years from 1920 to 1940 as the era of epidemics, in which high fertility was matched by high morbidity and mortality, and population levels fluctuated wildly. Medical institutions had minimal influence on this pattern.[52] The few impulsive individuals who were moved to intervene where they were needed and welcomed, were neither supported nor even observed, for a quarter of a century. If amateurishness and incompetence were criminal offences, then Australian colonialism in Papua would be profoundly guilty.

5
The political economy of health in
New Guinea between the wars

On the face of it, New Guinea should have developed a more effective medical service than Papua. It was the first theatre of military operations for Australian troops in the Great War, and a substantial garrison remained until the Armistice. The plantation economy had been developed by German entrepreneurs into a genuinely profitable industry, which was then expropriated and distributed among Australian ex-servicemen, who also enjoyed preferential appointment to the sizeable peace-time public service. From 1914 onwards, therefore, the Australian Government paid it much more attention than Papua enjoyed. Then the 1930s were dominated by the growth of a great gold mining industry in the eastern fringe of the highlands, on a much greater scale than any enterprise in Papua; and it was from New Guinea that most of the highlands exploration was launched. Again, as a conquest state governed by ex-soldiers, its expatriate population was larger and more articulate and united than that of the sister dependency.

New Guinea was held under a League of Nations Mandate, and it provided a major new responsibility for the small federal bureaucracy, which had to share responsibility for most other functions, with the constituent states of the Australian Commonwealth. The mandated territory assumed particular significance for Australian health planners. The Commonwealth Constitution gave the federal government scant authority over the states in matters of health. There was no federal Department of Health – only a quarantine section with limited powers, directed by Dr J.H.L. Cumpston.[1] In March 1921, however, Cumpston and the Rockefeller Foundation persuaded the federal government to create a separate Department of Health, with Cumpston as its Director-General. Tropical health was a decisive argument in this battle, because its field clearly transcended state boundaries, and because the federal government (rather than the individual states) was responsible for public health in the mandated territory. One of the very few institutions operated by the federal Department of Health was the Australian Institute of Tropical Medicine in Townsville, which therefore assumed a higher profile in the Health Department than we might otherwise expect. Cumpston placed effective allies in the few posts within his patronage: Dr J.S.C. Elkington as Director of Quarantine, and a young ex-serviceman Dr Raphael Cilento as Director of the Institute in Townsville.[2] He was thwarted in the appointment of the

Director of Health in New Guinea until 1924, when Cilento was commissioned to report on New Guinea Health services, and remained there as Director until 1928, self-consciously as Cumpston's agent.

Cumpston and his allies projected an ambitious 'Inland and Island Tropical Health Service' which would serve (and link) tropical northern Australia and the island territories, and an 'Austral-Pacific Regional Zone' of tight quarantine control, connecting the Australian, British and French dependencies of the south west Pacific. Although the 'South West Pacific (Quarantine) Zone' was agreed by the colonial powers only in 1928, its substance was approved at an international health conference held in Melbourne towards the end of 1926, which nominated Australia as the central administrative authority for the region.[3] It was at this late stage that Cumpston changed his strategy. In order to consolidate the new Department of Health in the federal bureaucracy, he switched his efforts away from tropical questions to the problems of urban, temperate Australia – where the great majority of electors lived.[4] In 1930 the Institute of Tropical Medicine was closed in tropical Townsville and re-located in temperate Sydney. Nevertheless New Guinea had been well endowed during the previous decade, with a Commonwealth Laboratory in Rabaul; and the quarantine network remained, requiring the regular reporting of infectious diseases, and encouraging medical authorities to meet at conferences and to keep in touch with each other.[5] Some regional research projects were promoted, pooling the scientific expertise of the colonial powers in the area.[6]

This network had little substance, but as an idea it persisted well into the 1930s. When Cilento became the coordinator of Australian medical research and programmes within the Tropical Hygiene branch of the Department of Health, the *Pacific Islands Monthly* expected him to be 'liaison officer between the medical men in the different tropical territories, in their war against disease'.[7] But Cilento's abrasive character created as much friction as cooperation. When he was appointed to report on health conditions in the Pacific, in 1928, Lieutenant-Governor Murray took strong exception

> I wish to protest against the appointment of Dr Cilento on the grounds of personal prejudice and of the probability that his investigation and his report would not be free of bias.[8]

Medical authorities continued to report to each other, through Australia and via the League of Nations offices in Geneva; but no new forms of organisation or control emerged, and the federal health bureaucracy downgraded its tropical responsibilities.

Although inter-territorial cooperation came to little, New Guinea's administration itself had great internal coherence. The territory remained under military occupation until 1921, and the garrison ethos survived the 20 years of peace. German planters and other property-owners were expropriated, and their properties sold to Australian ex-servicemen.[9] Every Administrator was either a serving military officer or an ex-officer; ex-servicemen were preferred in every administrative position, so that every Director of Health was an ex-serviceman and so were almost all the medical personnel. It was the shared experience of service under arms, which gave the new expatriate population its common values.

The Tropical Force, which garrisoned New Guinea until the end of the war, replaced the German doctors and nurses as soon as possible, and used military discipline to control malaria and dysentery – whereas the civilian expatriates were more relaxed in their medical measures.[10] The withdrawal of the garrison threw medical administration (as well as every other aspect of government) into brief disarray. Colonel Honman stayed on as Principal Medical Officer: when the Rockefeller hookworm crusade brought Lambert to the administrative centre at Rabaul, he found Honman to be

> a hard-crusted, soft-hearted old regular [and] all he knew about tropical medicine was what he had learned as personal physician to Prime Minister Billy Hughes. He wasn't afraid of liquor or anything else.[11]

There was a moment of acute alarm when smallpox entered across the uncontrolled border with Dutch New Guinea.[12] But a more persistent problem for medical administrators was the existence of two medical administrations. The Expropriation Board, which took charge of ex-enemy property until it could be transferred to Australian owners, had its own medical service, parallel to that of the administration. Responsibility was awkwardly divided, and resources inefficiently deployed.[13]

Cilento returned in 1924 to clean up the mess. His instincts were to develop the military values of his staff. He believed that

> the conditions in a native country are closely akin to those that must obtain during a military campaign [except that] the medical sanitary officer in New Guinea is dealing with irresponsible natives.[14]

As Maddocks pointed out later, Cilento and his successors ran the medical administration like an army. Cilento advised his staff that

> an officer's retention and promotion in this service will depend upon his knowledge, efficiency, loyalty to professional ideas, obedience to orders, careful observance of Acts, Regulations, Ordinances and instructions, and the constant exercise of discipline, sobriety, industry and good order.[15]

If medical personnel were the officers and other ranks of the organisation, how were they to deal with New Guineans?

1 Maintain a quiet manner and never lose temper.
2 Be insistent as to obedience in all details. Never pass over a neglect of duty, however small.
3 Maintain reserve with natives. Do not chat with them about matters outside work. Never joke with them.
4 Be as considerate as possible, but never weak.

5 Never forget a promise, nor make one which you may not be able to keep.[16]

This was not a bedside manner; nor can we imagine Strong, his head full of anthropology and recipes, issuing such edicts in Papua.

Cilento had such a clear vision of how his staff should behave, that he could almost be considered the first medical strategist since MacGregor. When technical issues came to his attention, he grasped their political significance. One vexed issue of the 1920s was whether or not Melanesians should be encouraged (or indeed permitted) to wear European clothes:

> Clothes were worn for decoration long before they were worn for decency, and such is still the case among all ranks and all colours. They add to self-respect and self-esteem. Psychologically, this is of the utmost value to a subject race. An absolute prohibition against clothing would be recognised by the natives as a barrier that places them definitely and finally in the position of obvious inferiority. Inferiority there doubtless is, but its ostentation, however unintentional, is harmful and unnecessary.[17]

He had an equally clear view of the political purpose of medical services to New Guineans:

> Medical officers on patrol are requested to confine their attentions as much as possible in new districts to the enhancing of the prestige of Australian medicine. They are required first to win the confidence of the people and to map the distribution of disease ... Having won the confidence of the natives, and in process of so doing, they are advised to treat all cases in which there is a chance of a spectacular and ready cure, e.g. the infant of a chieftain may be treated for framboesia ... By following this process of opportunism, there comes finally a time when the villagers learn to have the greatest respect for, and belief in, the curative powers of the medical officer.[18]

Cilento was not quite a medical strategist: his vision did not encompass the field of health and illness beyond the army which he led, except to command the respect and confidence of the conquered population. There were, for instance, no 'chieftains' in New Guinea, nor would there be any great resistance to medical officers once news of the yaws treatment percolated through the villages. Equally, the structure of the medical service made nonsense of dogmatic centralism. In Rabaul, 'officers' and 'other ranks' of the administration socialised in separate clubs; and the dispersed centres of government were rarely visited by headquarters staff, so that Stan Christian – a medical assistant from 1922 until war broke out again – never met a Director of Health.[19] The daily tasks of a doctor in charge of a district, let alone an Assistant on patrol from clinic to aid-post, imposed a rhythm quite impervious to the instructions coming from Rabaul.

There was another source of suggestions on medical strategy during the 1920s. During the transition from German to Australian ownership, most plantation production was taken over by a single agency, the Expropriation Board. Its chief executive officer was Walter Lucas, an experienced employee of Burns, Philp & Co., the island trading firm, and a confidant of Prime Minister Hughes.[20] When Lucas spoke, the Australian Government listened. He had better-developed ideas about medical policy than any other representative of the plantation industry, and he stated them in 1922

> It is beyond dispute that ... the planter must think not only for today, but must give considerable thought to the future ... the planter has the strongest motives of self-interest in assisting substantially any measures undertaken for the amelioration and eradication of tropical diseases, including research ... and in the proper organisation of medical staffs.
>
> Such measures are not only necessary to prevent the native race dying out, [but also allow] an increase in population which is essential to meet the future requirements of the industries.

Lucas conceded that, if planters were well established, it would be proper to levy them to establish a medical service. Acting as trustee for planters collectively, the Expropriation Board was willing to grant £10,000 to this purpose.[21] The grant was not conditional, but in a later memo Lucas described the kinds of investment which he thought appropriate. The hospitals inherited from the German administration were more numerous and better equipped than those in Papua, so Lucas considered them quite satisfactory for the foreseeable future. Instead of building hospitals, the new medical service should concentrate on rural health, and give more weight to preventive than to curative medicine.[22]

As it happened, the Director of Health put forward his own proposal at almost the same time, and its elements were quite different from those which Lucas envisaged:

Instruments	£	1,500
Equipment and bedding		2,000
European hospitals		1,250
Native hospitals		1,500
Drugs and dressings		2,250
Medical staff and transport		1,500
		————
Total	£	10,000

A medical schooner – costing about £1,500 – was to be provided from some other source.[23] Lucas's demand for a labourer-centred medical strategy was simply drowned out in a welter of competing claims, each of them technically defensible, but adding up to a medical service of a quite different kind. The rival claims arose from the experience and professional interests of the medical officers, not from analysis of the New Guinea situation. Lucas might have sustained his campaign, had opportunity offered. However, the logistics of valuing the expropriated properties, organising their sale and transferring ownership, proved clumsy; and by the late 1920s, when the process was complete, the plantation industry was plunged into financial crisis and fragmented into individual plantations with no clear voice in public policy.[24] The Annual Report for 1921–22 stated flatly that £10,000 from the Expropriation Board had been spent on 'the improvement of hospital accommodation, and the purchase of additional supplies of instruments etc'.

The consequence was muddle. Civil administration, launched in 1921, set itself medical goals; three years later Cilento judged that none of them had been met. Racial segregation was not yet complete, the government ignored its own housing regulations and standards, and neither hygiene nor sanitation was satisfactory. He blamed four general circumstances: the lack of personnel trained in tropical conditions, shortage of funds, a general unconcern with preventive medicine, and squabbling between departments (exacerbated by the independence of the Expropriation Board). In 59 pages of text, weighted by statistical appendices, Cilento condemned most individuals and institutions in the mandated territory.[25]

The organisation did improve, as ordinary conditions replaced war-time emergency. During the 1920s, between 10 and 14 doctors were deployed; and by the end of the 1930s there were 22, many of whom had attended courses at Townsville (or at Sydney, where the institute was transferred in 1930).[26] From the base hospitals, each doctor supervised the work of European medical assistants, who patrolled the countryside, and of hospital orderlies. Some medical assistants were in effect doctors: they built small hospitals of bush materials, they gave injections, and they performed surgery when no doctor was available.[27] The German institution of medical *tultuls* persisted in the villages. Dr Jackson at Kavieng reported on the fairly newly-trained *tultuls* in New Ireland in 1922. They had received six weeks' instruction in dressing wounds.

> The main idea has been to instruct the tultuls in the recognition and not so much the treatment of disease and so far they have done well all that was expected of them.[28]

Other doctors at other base hospitals entertained different expectations of a *tultul*. He was often the only villager familiar with simple English (the use of *tok pisin* was not encouraged), so he was often absent from the village acting as a court interpreter. However, he was very useful to the patrolling medical assistants, who knew that there would be a named official to meet at the end of a day's march. By the end of the 1930s there were over 4,000 medical *tultuls*.[29]

During the 1920s the medical services covered only the coastal regions and the islands of the Bismarck Archipelago, a zone of plantations and small-holder production. During the 1920s, Lutheran and Catholic missionaries and evangelists began to work in the eastern highlands, but they kept quiet about their discoveries.[30] During the 1930s, however, gold miners ventured into the highlands, and missionaries, administrators and prospectors met the unexpectedly dense population of the inland region. On the one hand, this stretched medical resources; on the other hand the mining revenue was a welcome supplement. In any case, the Depression made doctors and medical assistants more willing to take jobs outside Australia.[31] The most alarming medical consequence of 'opening up' the highlands was the revelation of a large population highly susceptible to malaria and tuberculosis, to which they would necessarily be exposed. The favourable impression made by the good health of the highlanders was tinged by a sense of their vulnerability.[32]

New Guinea's medical administration was certainly more professional than Papua's. Cilento conducted demographic research (though he may have cut corners in doing so).[33] And Rabaul had a Commonwealth government laboratory, with trained staff, attracting regular visits by specialists from Townsville and Sydney.[34] After the entry of smallpox early in the 1920s, there were few breaches of the quarantine cordon. (When a doctor's child returned from leave in Australia, bringing infectious measles, evading quarantine, and starting an epidemic, the doctor was required to resign.[35]) Nevertheless tuberculosis made steady progress in the Melanesian population, and venereal disease was a persistent problem (especially in New Ireland) despite draconian controls.[36]

Curiously, this impressively regimented service and its large numbers of qualified practitioners offered much the same pattern of treatment for most of the population as in amateurish Papua. During 1925–26, for instance

> specific campaigns have been continued against Framboesia and Hookworm disease. There has been instituted a considerable campaign against Gonorrhoea, while strong representations have been made to Central Administration on the question of diet deficiencies and the prevention of beri-beri. These four diseases, practically speaking, have absorbed the energies of the Department from the point of view of field campaigns.[37]

That emphasis persisted. During 1938–39, medical patrols gave 37,467 yaws injections, 5,277 hookworm treatments, 10,099 'minor' treatments, and sent 2,656 people to hospital.[38]

To combat infection on plantations, a complex structure of control was placed on paper, requiring plantation managers to provide health care in proportion to the size of the labour force. However

> in 1925, when several hundred [people] suffering from venereal disease were placed in concentration camps at Rabaul and Kavieng for treatment, an unexpected failure in the supplies of fresh food produced an almost immediate outbreak of beri-beri . . . The disease occurred earlier and more severely in the case of indentured natives who had been living upon store rations and engaged in regular daily labour, than in those brought in from villages, though in each instance, the nutritional defence level was lower than might have been expected . . . At that particular time the diet that was official for natives . . . was absolutely lacking in vitamins of any kind whatever.[39]

It seems unlikely that an administration, which could not prevent nutritional disease in its own facilities, had much impact on the nutrition and general health of the plantation labour force. Yaws and hookworm eradication, even if they had been effective, were a distraction from tasks which a medical service could have accomplished, relying upon public health knowledge instead of concentrating on 'tropical' infections.

Medical possibilities were subordinated to social and political circumstances, to a quite remarkable degree. A clear instance of this constraint was the refusal to train New Guineans to take part in the medical service (see chapter 6). Another constraint had to do with sex. Cilento warned: 'Curious situations occasionally develop (as in West Fiji) when black men are the only available practitioners for white women'.[40] His sensibility in matters of race and gender did not encourage him to ask what curious situations might develop when there was no medical practitioner at all. The opposite situation – white women doctors or nurses tending black men – was not allowed to occur either in New Guinea or in Papua. Women could apply for positions as doctors, but they were never appointed – even in one case where a competent woman doctor was the only applicant.[41] Dr Phyllis Cilento, who accompanied her husband to New Guinea, evidently practised only among the New Guinea Chinese community.[42] One consequence of this blinkering network of taboos was to draw a veil over high maternal mortality rates. Medical assistants (especially if they learned their trade during the war) had no expertise in treating the 'peculiar complaints' of women, and a female patient might be turned away from treatment if she were found to be pregnant.[43]

As the expatriate population increased through the 1920s, and officers were allowed to bring their wives and children to the mandated territory, an articulate group of women brought their needs to the attention of the Administration:

> The nursing services of the Territory are confined at present to one institution – Namanula Hospital – which serves the [white] residents of Rabaul and District ... The hospital system still shows marked evidence of its military origin, and, up to the present [1926] its chief function has been the treatment of officials and their dependents ... On the other hand, owing to the increase of private citizens and the numbers of women and children ... there is a growing demand for increased work in child welfare, the pre-natal and post-natal education of mothers, district nursing etc.

The nursing service was reorganised to cope with the settlers' needs.[44]

In 1930 the Administration did open a clinic for New Guinean mothers and infants. On this occasion the planters and the *Pacific Islands Monthly* protested about spending money on non-labourers; but the more serious difficulty was to recruit nurses who were willing to live at the clinic centre. As in Papua therefore, all maternal and child health services became the province of the missions.[45] Only the missions could attract and retain people willing to work with New Guineans, in village conditions. The missions therefore provided the bulk of those medical services to the rural population.

Relations between church and state were regularised at a conference in 1926. It was agreed that the missions should provide services ancillary to those of the administration, yet they would not come under the control of the Health Department. On medical policy, the conference agreed that:

> natives be encouraged to value drugs and services, and eventually to pay for them, but meanwhile to make a token payment;
>
> that village committees be encouraged, and directed towards sanitation;
>
> that a high birthrate be maintained, by discouraging contraception, abortion and infanticide, and by providing midwives and improved food supplies;
>
> and that clothing restrictions were not beneficial.[46]

Since the aims of church and state were much the same, there was no need for government control. In practice, the New Guinean service closely resembled that of Papua. Both were concerned about depopulation, both considered the missions best equipped to deal with that question, and in both cases the enduring crisis of high maternal mortality rates was disregarded. The Papuan administration offered a baby bounty (to men) to sustain high birth rates while the New Guinea administration relied more heavily on criminal sanctions against birth control. In each case the maternal and child health service evolved overwhelmingly as a child-care service, offering only occasional ad hoc assistance to the process of motherhood.

The administration of New Guinea between the wars stands out in the history of Australian governments, as the most sustained experiment in military rule. So marked was the militarist style of government, that its values (including a sharp differentiation between men and women, and an inviolable separation of the conquering and the conquered population) over-rode everything else. Further, the application of military measures to the regulation of plantation labour (instead of the well-argued programme which Lucas proposed) proved counter-productive.

At the same time, the technical achievements of medicine (especially the use of novarsenobillon against yaws, and the belief that oil of chemopodium would drive out hookworm) diverted medical resources into the elimination of specific infections. These campaigns had one immense attraction: they lent themselves to statistical precision. And they had several immense disadvantages: they were ineffectual, they were of marginal significance to the population's health even when they were well executed, and they distracted attention from other measures which were technically possible and medically advisable. What could have been done, and what was being done in Australia, was not done in New Guinea: the regulation of diet, the provision of clean water and nutritious food, and the isolation of such non-tropical infectious diseases as tuberculosis. New Guineans could have been healthier in 1939 than they had ever been before:

instead, they were exposed to a wider variety of infections, and those who entered the commercial economy were especially vulnerable because of living conditions and diets which reduced their resistance to infection of any kind. In both dependencies, colonialism was literally a health hazard.

The limitations of the political economy approach in understanding health policies and programmes should now be apparent. The structure of New Guinea's colonial economy was a plantation system in the 1920s, supplemented and largely superceded by a mining economy during the 1930s: in each phase, it was desirable to increase the indigenous population, to ensure the health and strength of the indentured labour force, and to direct medical resources towards preventive health measures. This is substantially the strategy which Lucas advocated on behalf of the managers of the plantation economy. In practice, neither the Australian Government nor the mandated territory's administration insisted that this strategy be adopted by the Health Department. Instead, first Honman and then Cilento devised policies in the light of their professional interests and instincts. The outcome was a series of policies and programmes which were couched in a stridently militarist rhetoric, but whose substance resembled those in neighbouring Papua – which had neither a healthy plantation economy nor a substantial mining sector between the wars.

If policies were not determined by the colonial state to meet the needs of capital, where did they come from? One important but diffuse source was the social imperatives of colonialism itself, in territories very recently brought under settler control and still somewhat resembling conquest states. The colonists' survival was an absolute priority. When the colonists were more secure, they remained a tiny minority whose control was frail, and whose prestige alone seemed to guarantee their survival and authority. These considerations help explain the otherwise irrational insistence that white female nurses should tend only white patients, and the priority given to medicating the small expatriate society. Within these constraints, doctors were further blinkered by the mental strait-jacket of tropical medicine, which specified only a limited number of diseases and complaints which required the attention of tropical doctors.

6
Medical education

The early medical authorities in colonial Papua – whose own life expectancy was a matter of nervous doubt – had no opportunity to teach each other nor to instruct Papuans. Breinl's visit from the Institute of Tropical Medicine encouraged Strong's interest in the bowel parasites of plantation workers,[1] but the official record makes no reference to formal teaching. Informally, though, doctors encouraged settlers to take their bitter quinine regularly, and through the *Handbook on the treatment and prevention of disease in Papua when medical advice is unobtainable*[2] (that is, for most of the people, most of the time) to dress wounds, purge fevers, and remain cheerful. The hookworm campaign involved a programme of lectures on personal hygiene in Lambert's idiosyncratic pidgin, and government patrols encouraged the building (and use) of pit latrines, and discouraged traditions of allowing corpses to decompose in villages.

Their German counterparts were better equipped to embark on an educational programme, and in the few years before the Great War a number of *heil tultuls* received a few weeks' instruction in hospitals, before they returned to their villages.[3] The vaccination programmes had an educational dimension as well; although some missionaries intruded more theology than therapy into their advice.[4] The innovation of *heil tultuls* was one of very few German ideas to survive the transition to Australian rule:

> This training [as 'medical *tultuls*'] consists of teaching how to dress and treat tropical sores and other diseases, the recognition of cases requiring hospital treatment, administering treatment ordered by medical officers under the supervision of European medical assistants, assisting at operations, elementary rules of sanitation and the methods of quarantining infectious or contagious cases etc. When they are considered efficient, they are given the position of medical tultul and returned to their village with a supply of drugs and dressings ... and are given a cap with a Red Cross band on it. A patrol goes out about every three months and inspects the medical supplies and the progress made by these medical tultuls ... With lengthy training they become most efficient as hospital orderlies, dressing wounds, assisting at operations and post mortems and they learn to administer drugs intravenously. Their efficiency is undoubted, and their keenness in learning most evident.[5]

The Department's enthusiasm for *tultuls* was tempered during the next decade or so, and they were deployed almost entirely in villages, where supervision and inspection were irregular. By 1938–39 there were 4,003 in

New Guinea. Medical patrols led by doctors or medical assistants were able to visit only 1,885 villages in that year, so only 1,519 of the *tultuls* were inspected. 17 per cent of these inspected were described as poor in their work, and the same percentage had their supplies in a poor condition.[6] Since a medical patrol was always preceded by a good warning through the bush telegraph,[7] it is rather surprising that so many *tultuls* were caught unprepared.

The training and supervision of *tultuls* in Australian New Guinea was matched by a more general scheme of in-service training for European medical assistants, who were encouraged to study for examinations leading to promotion. Whenever a medical assistant was stationed at a hospital with a resident doctor, that preparation could be quite rigorous.[8] There was also provision for a handful of medical assistants to study formally at the University of Sydney. Doctors, on the other hand, were encouraged to take a short course at the Institute of Tropical Medicine if they had no previous exposure to the techniques of tropical medicine.[9]

When the Depression struck the territories, it spurred medical planners to explore the greater use of Melanesians, if only because their wages were so much lower than those of Australians. Strong of Papua made the running. During the 1920s, he had trained Papuans to administer bismuth injections against yaws, to hand out doses against tinea, and to give 'simple medical and surgical treatment'. By 1932 it was clear that better use should and could be made of Papuan medical workers. While Strong was on leave in Sydney that year, he discussed the matter with the Minister for Health (who was also Minister for Territories), Cumpston the Director-General of Health, and Harvey Sutton the Director of the School of Public Health and Tropical Medicine. They agreed to cooperate in 'giving Papuan medical students some training in the subjects of the first and second M.B. examinations'.[10] A scheme along these lines came into operation during 1933.

The decision to train students at Sydney was a decision not to send them to Fiji. Dr Sam Lambert had tired of the hookworm crusade, and thrown his considerable energy into the Central Medical School in Suva, which trained 'Native Medical Practitioners' to serve in most of the islands of the central Pacific. From Suva he wrote to his old friend Dr Tom Brennan, now Director of Public Health in Rabaul:

> These Native Medical Practitioners are just the thing needed in Papua and New Guinea. The longer I am out here the surer I am that the answer to many problems not alone of medicine but of administration also is to teach natives to care for their own kind ... The Government and missions here should take young ones in hand early and get them ready for the school here.[11]

Brennan responded by proposing a medical school in Rabaul itself, consisting of two sections:

> A senior class of a few intelligent half-castes ... [and a] junior class of intelligent, partly educated, native youths – about 16 years old – who have

been selected from Administration and Mission Schools ... [With] my
experience of what can be achieved with the very small, but rapidly growing,
minority of intelligent natives (even houseboys), I would predict that the
system of trial and error (with error much in the foreground in the beginning –
but visually receding year by year) will eventually (with patience, and with a
definite final object in view), result in a Native Medical Service.[12]

The Administrator was much taken by the scheme, which he forwarded to
Canberra where it was sent to the Director-General of Health for his
observations. It was here that the proposal foundered.

Director-General Cumpston discussed the question with Strong, and
with Cilento (who was briefly Cumpston's deputy). Cumpston and Strong
believed that

any attempt to create quasi-medical men would be a mistake, that it is far
better to concentrate on the training of the natives to an increasingly efficient
form of first aid work, gradually attaining to a point comparable to that of a
male nurse or hospital orderly in the army.[13]

It was at this point that Strong developed his own scheme for training
primary-school leavers as Papuan medical assistants. Cilento's response was
much more damning:

The ideal in New Guinea and allied territories, owing to the low stage of
civilization and the absence of social organisation amongst the natives, is to
build up a subsidiary and auxiliary service of native medical orderlies who may
by a process of training and elimination extending over a generation, finally
result in making available a number of fully trained native medical practitioners. These will function amongst selected village communities of natives,
who during the same generation have become accustomed to the idea of the
local native as a minor medical authority, and to western medicine as natural
and desirable ... The American attempt at medical penetration throughout
the whole of the Western Pacific is based upon the high organisation of the
Polynesian and semi-Polynesian races. It is inapplicable to New Guinea.
    The training at Suva is entirely in English: the products of the training
... are poor, lacking in initiative, with some medical learning by [illegible]
only and temperamental disabilities that necessitate constant supervision.[14]

The Administrator, General Griffith, knew only that Melanesians
from the New Hebrides and the Solomon Islands had successfully graduated
from the Central Medical School, and he was not impressed by the
arguments against New Guinean educational capacity. However

Two such eminent Medical Officers as Drs Cumpston and Cilento having
pronounced against the scheme, it would be presumptuous on my part to offer
any further suggestion ... therefore it is with the very greatest reluctance and
grief that I drop the scheme.[15]

Griffith was not alone in his grief. The *Pacific Islands Monthly*, never an
advocate of opportunities for Pacific Islanders, still complained that

there seems to be no policy under which medical work is controlled and
directed. Other territories have successfully instituted a system of training

> Native Medical Practitioners ... The New Guinea administration has done
> nothing beyond imparting a little medical training to native hospital assist-
> ants.[16]

In this instance at least, the bigotry of Australian professional men
exceeded that of the planters.

Meanwhile Strong brought together a dozen candidates for a preliminary course. Some were already working in the department; others were
selected by the missionary Percy Chatterton from the brightest boys in
Hanuabada primary school; all were Hanuabadans who had to be fully
literate in Motu, have some knowledge of English, and possess some simple
arithmetic. Strong taught them himself, in Motu and English, for the few
months between their selection and their departure for Sydney.[17]

In Sydney, the young men were hermetically insulated against acci-
dental social contacts:

> At Manly the Papuans are excellently accommodated in the premises origi-
> nally built for the accommodation of seamen suffering from venereal disease
> ... Mr E. H. Adams, a European Medical Assistant, resides at Manly with
> the Papuans, accompanies them to and from the University each day, and
> exercises an immediate supervision ... The Papuans have a large ward to live
> in and the option of using another room. They are provided with two Papuan
> cook boys, who do the cooking and keep the quarters clean ... It saves
> expense and renders it easy to control them and to keep possible undesirable
> influences away from them. At the University Dr Clements [their personal
> tutor] has a first class lecture room with laboratory equipment ... The
> Papuans also have the use of a room for themselves during the lunch hour with
> excellent lavatory accommodation available. They also have facilities for
> boiling water for the making of tea during the lunch hour.[18]

Having excluded all possible distractions, Strong organised an occasional controlled excursion, to play cricket, to attend church, or (courtesy of
New South Wales railways) to the bush to observe procedures for a railway
accident. The curriculum which Clements taught included anatomy,
weights and measures, physics and chemistry, physiology and some elemen-
tary medical and surgical procedures. Strong explained in Motu on Satur-
days, anything they had not grasped in English. And 20 weeks later they
were shipped home.[19]

This was an impressive pedagogical feat, which allowed for the
minimal formal education which the young men had received, and which
equipped them to fulfil the limited procedures of the Papuan medical
programme. It was repeated the following year, and the year after, before
settler unease at Papuans' presumed exposure to the flesh pots of Sydney
brought the experiment to an end.[20]

The educational programme can hardly be faulted for what it
achieved. More serious was the opportunity lost. One of Strong's objections
to Fiji was the need to send Papuans away from home for four years, which
he reckoned was much longer than they would tolerate. But the penalty for

a strictly controlled programme was the narrowness of the expertise acquired. The young men became dispensers or well-trained nurses, but not doctors. And when Strong retired, and the Pacific War ushered in a quite new era of therapies, most of the Papuan medical assistants were lost to the medical profession.[21]

Not only were all the trainees Hanuabadans: they were all male. The bachelor Strong was never able to focus his attention on women, and certainly no female companionship gave him as much satisfaction as his friendships in the Papuan administration, or with his Papuan proteges. He was content to delegate the care of women and children to the missions, as we have seen.[22] It was not in his muddled good nature to dismiss the possibility of teaching women as definitively as Cilento, who decreed that 'attempts to institute services, either white or black, in this regard must be futile at present owing to the status of women in native tribes, the religious and other restrictions surrounding the act of birth, etc., etc'.[23] In both New Guinea and Papua, the missions simply taught women to nurse and to be midwives, without stopping to worry about quasi-anthropological objections.

In both dependencies, then, the provision of medical education reflected the fantasies of a small expatriate population surrounded by villagers whose lives were but dimly perceived through a miasma of racist and sexist stereotypes, and whose capacities were neither tested nor significantly stretched. The fact that those few Melanesians who were offered any opportunity whatever – medical *tultuls* in New Guinea, Papuan medical assistants, and Kwato community nurses – responded eagerly and successfully to their new careers, should make us recognise the scale of the opportunity lost.

7

The Pacific War: the condition of the people

The military imagery which coloured medical discussions in New Guinea between the wars reflected Australia's traumatic tradition as supplier of shock-troops for the British Empire. Yet the Pacific War caught the Australian government unprepared. Military planners certainly expected a world war – but a re-run of the Great War. The troops were equipped to fight on the Western Front, but were actually sent to North Africa and to the Middle East, which had been a sideshow in the Great War. The soldiers were equipped badly for the North African desert, and not at all for New Guinea.[1] Some had been despatched to Malaya, lest the Japanese join in the war. When Singapore fell, and Japanese forces swept through the western Pacific to occupy the Bismarck Archipelago in January 1942, most Australian troops were either committed in the Middle East or captured in South East Asia. Only the tiny garrisons in Rabaul and Port Moresby had direct experience of jungle conditions.[2] Between 1942 and 1945, the brutal fighting in the Solomons and New Guinea would be won by those armies best able to maintain their fighting strength in enervating temperatures and humidity, beset by endemic malaria and epidemic dysentery.

Japan entered the Pacific War with every advantage of experience. As early as 1904, during their war against Russia, they had demonstrated that military discipline could restrict non-battle casualties.[3] Since the early 1930s, their armies had been deployed abroad in Manchuria and China: their medical officers had experienced every environmental and logistical problem. That advantage was soon lost in New Guinea. Supplies were interdicted once the army was isolated from Japan so there were no more drugs or dressings after 1942. Perhaps the chief medical hazard was malaria. Post-war investigators found that Japanese soldiers were particularly highly infected, and suffered a very high mortality rate. They laid some of the blame at the door of medical officers, who were not using 'standard or proven methods' of treatment.[4]

There was another element in their tragedy. Sir William Refshauge explained the link between morale and mortality:

> In war-time, a highly disciplined force, with good morale and good leadership, simply doesn't get sick (except from things like appendicitis, which can't be helped); but low morale and loose discipline quickly produce illness.[5]

58

Once the Japanese forces were isolated, their future held only a lingering defeat, and morale collapsed. During the long and bitter retreat, the soldiers 'left evidence of dysenteric infection, in their fouling of the ground, for their hygiene was primitive'.[6] By the last months of the war, Japanese casualties outnumbered Australian by at least ten to one.[7] Japan may have lost 150,000 men in New Guinea.[8]

Australian troops also lost the advantage of their experience in the Great War. Summing up the hard-won experience of the earlier Tropical Force in Rabaul, the official historian declared:

> never again, in a fight against the attacks of a treacherous tropical climate . . . will an Australian administration be handicapped to the same extent as was the military administration in New Guinea.[9]

His prediction was falsified. Brigadier Disher arrived in Port Moresby at the end of November, 1942, to find that 'all people from forward seem to have malaria'. His visit to the front confirmed his impression. When he took over in December as Deputy Director Military Services for New Guinea Force, he found the hospitals overflowing. The sick and wounded could neither be discharged nor repatriated to Australia; under the beds were stretchers, and all were occupied. He believed the situation would become worse, because supplies (including quinine) were inadequate for the Milne Bay campaign.[10]

The first Allied victory against Japanese land forces was achieved at Milne Bay in 1942 and was partly the result of fortunate timing:

> At the end of December [1942] the malarial incidence rate, which had reached 33 per thousand per week in September (1,716 per thousand per year) rose to 82 per thousand per week (4,264 per thousand per year): at this rate the force would have fallen to zero in three months. During the third week of December 1,083 out of 12,000 men contracted malaria . . . in the last few months of 1942 malaria was coming to be regarded with an air of inevitability . . .
>   It was fortunate that the brief campaign had come so early, otherwise the saturation of the force by malaria would have been a serious drawback to the success of those sharp conflicts which turned back the Japanese.[11]

Two factors enabled Australian and American troops to survive endemic malaria. One was already known from the Great War: ruthless discipline. By the end of the Pacific War, troops were dosed daily, under an officer's inspection: they were required to use mosquito nets, and to keep themselves covered. Malaria could eventually be considered as a self-inflicted wound.[12] The second factor was the new prophylactic drug, atebrin. Atebrin was known before the war, and a handful of doctors had faith in it.[13] When the Japanese occupation of the Dutch East Indies interrupted supplies of quinine, atebrin had to be used instead: the problem was uncertainty about appropriate dosages. Applied research in north Queensland, organised by Brigadier Hamilton Fairley, determined correct dosage, and the research results were presented to military commanders with some force.[14]

Table 2

Casualty	1914–18 war	1939–45 war
Gross strength of force	416,809	727,703
Number who served overseas	331,781	396,661
Battle casualty deaths	53,993	18,713
Wounded in action	137,013	22,116
Total battle casualties	212,773	61,575
Non-battle casualty deaths	6,291	6,038
Sick outside Australia	393,155	433,587
Overall total of casualties	616,606	534,596
Mortality from all causes	60,284 (1 in 7)	24,751 (1 in 30)

During the Australian retreat along the Kokoda Track, not only malaria, but also respiratory infections and exhaustion sapped the soldiers' strength. Soon 'diarrhoea was almost universal', followed swiftly by true dysentery. Once the dispersed forces were concentrated, and hygiene discipline could be re-imposed, the diarrhoea abated. The decisive weapon against that, and against dysentery, was sulphaguanadine, the first of the new 'miracle drugs' to be deployed in the New Guinea campaign. Other medical hazards – scrub typhus among them – were tackled through dedicated research and fierce discipline.[15] There is much force in Refshauge's view that 'we won the war because we beat malaria, and scrub typhus, and dysentery':[16] but it had been a close run thing.

The far-reaching significance and impact of changing medical conditions, is best shown by comparing casualties in the two World Wars[17] (see table 2).

Compared to soldiers in the Great War, soldiers in the Second World War were much more numerous; but fewer of them fell ill. More went overseas, but fewer were killed in action; they were much less likely to be wounded in action, and the survival rate (from illness as well as from wounds) rose dramatically. If we omitted the morbidity and mortality of Australians as prisoners of war, who had little access to drugs or doctors, the contrast would be even more arresting.

The impact of the war on the health of Papua New Guineans is not quantifiable in the same way. In order to assess it, we need to remind ourselves of the structure of every-day life on the outbreak of war. Almost all Papua New Guineans lived in villages or hamlets: the plantations and gold mining enclaves certainly drew their labour force from the countryside, but the ordinary pattern of employment was to recruit young men from village communities for a year or two, under indenture. Food production continued without interruption, since young men were the least productive members of rural society, and could be spared for a couple of years without serious consequence. The war made much greater demands on the population than they had endured in peace-time. In areas controlled by the Allies and by the Japanese, men were recruited not only for the armed forces, but in much larger numbers as carriers and labourers, and for much longer periods of service.[18] Hanuabadans on the outskirts of Port Moresby were evacuated to villages along the coast: but even in villages which did not have to move, the massive recruitment of carriers disrupted production. Food production was left to women; quantities fell; and malnutrition was reported.[19] The recruits themselves received regular rations, but the old, the women, and the children left at home had to fend for themselves.

The area most seriously affected was the Gazelle peninsula in New Britain, the base for the largest Japanese force in the region, which remained more or less intact until the war ended in 1945. Cut off from external food supplies, Japanese and Tolai alike suffered acute hunger. The Japanese were largely protected from the daily bombing raids by an intricate network of tunnels; but the bombs played havoc with agriculture, and soldiers and civilians alike paid the price.[20] Almost all of coastal and island New Guinea, and the northern province of Papua, sustained heavy fighting for some months, with predictable disruption of food supplies.

Bearing in mind Cilento's observation, in the 1920s, that an unexpected interruption to the food supplies in government institutions produced widespread beri-beri,[21] the dislocation of the war predisposed the village people to a range of infections and debility. Furthermore, the relatively good health of the population rested still, in the 1940s, upon isolation from vectors of infection. That isolation was shattered by large-scale movements of soldiers and carriers and refugees. One potential disaster was successfully avoided. Highlanders were not recruited to work or carry in the low country, apart from a small number early in the war. A Native Labour Commission in New Guinea in 1939 had advised against recruiting above an altitude of 4,000 feet for coastal employment: medical advice (including that of Dr Carl Gunther who worked at Bulolo in the eastern fringe of the highlands) was unanimous that the risk was too great.[22] When war broke out, Stan Christian was sent to the highlands to confirm that malaria was absent: when he reported that this was the case, there was no recruitment.[23] Evidently 70 men had been brought from Simbu in the highlands to Lae on the coast in 1935, following the murder of two pioneer missionaries: after two months the District Officer had sent them home because they were suffering so intensely from malaria, which eventually killed 20 or 30 of them.[24] Despite the ban on war-time recruitment, some emergency seemed to justify the recruitment of 200 highlanders to work in Lae. By December 1945 they had all been repatriated – apart from half a dozen who remained in hospital.[25]

Highlanders were the only large group of people whose lives were not drastically upset by population movements. When civilian government broke down soon after the Japanese invasion, all isolated lepers, tuberculosis patients, and carriers of venereal diseases, dispersed to their homes.[26] Dysentery accompanied all troop movements. Epidemics broke out everywhere, even in the highlands.[27] In the highlands case, the rapid distribution of sulphaguanadine stemmed the outbreak; but there must have been many other epidemics, beyond the vision of the authorities, or beyond the range of drugs and careful nursing.

War not only introduced new risks: it removed old remedies. Doctors and nurses in New Guinea administration service or working for missions were mainly withdrawn when the invasion began. Those who did not withdraw in time, were killed or interned.[28] The Japanese authorities made no significant arrangements to protect the health of civilians within the areas they controlled. A handful of mission-trained New Guinean medical assistants remained at large, and bravely gave what treatment they could, from a dwindling supply of medicines and dressings;[29] but the medical *tultuls* had not been taught to cope with medical responsibilities beyond reporting. In Papua, medical personnel were also withdrawn, or drafted into the Australian New Guinea Administrative Unit (ANGAU) which began to build a civilian medical service. Since the prime responsibility of ANGAU was to provide carriers, and they operated as a military unit, their care for the civilian population was necessarily uneven. Army medical services were not normally available for civilians – army hospitals were mobile, and were moved intact when a military crisis passed. On occasion, military doctors did treat civilians, and provided drugs, but these occasions were exceptional.[30] In general, it was ANGAU which provided such health care as was available.

Jinks summarises ANGAU's annual report for 1944, and reaches this judgment:

> Although in 1944 ANGAU had only ten medical officers, compared with sixteen in the pre-war administration, it also employed 113 European medical assistants, compared with 49, and operated 53 hospitals, in comparison with 20. It is more difficult to compare performance, since statistics for ANGAU were compiled on a different basis from those for the civil medical service, but the sheer volume of ANGAU effort speaks for itself. In the year to September 1944, the medical service branch of the Unit treated 84,617 labourers and villagers in its hospitals and inspected 124,362 people during 523 patrols, administering treatment in 68,332 cases. The cost of medical equipment, drugs, rations and comforts in this period was more than £240,000 or 35% more than the whole budget of Papua in 1939/40.[31]

ANGAU officers certainly did as well as they could, but this may not have been enough to off-set the massively increased problems endured by the rural population. ANGAU was overwhelmingly a male organisation, primarily concerned with labour recruitment, and therefore as little con-cerned with women and children as the pre-war services. Although a large and complex establishment was put together, this was partly the product of ad hoc courses, a few weeks in duration, which transformed eager amateurs into medical assistants expected to perform tasks ordinarily entrusted to graduate doctors.[32] It was heroic medicine, on an unprecedented scale: but the medical conditions were acute, and even ANGAU was probably unable to restore the pre-war balance.

Introducing his study of *Clinical problems of war*, Walker points to the effect of each World War on the outlook of clinical medicine.[33] The Second War promoted the role of the miracle drugs. Penicillin was developed as a war measure, and spread widely via the Allied forces. Sulpha drugs had been invented before the war, but the rapid diffusion of sulphaguanadine (even into the New Guinea highlands) owed everything to military necessity. The proper use of atebrin, and a better understanding of quinine, also followed from war-time research. (Even tuberculosis, which had defied scientists for half a century, began to yield in the late 1940s.[34]) Secondly, the existence of these drugs transformed the nature of medical work. Whereas a dysentery patient in the 1930s could regain health only through careful nursing, that patient in the 1940s would respond directly to drugs. Medical education was transformed by shifts of this kind. Thirdly, the scope of medicine itself changed:

> Certainly we would never have conquered malaria, without enforcing the use of atebrin, whether people liked it or not ... There was the immunisation programme too, against typhoid; also against tetanus. Now we had no compunction about that. After the war ... the world-wide campaign against smallpox was similar. This all came from World War Two and the knowledge that if you didn't do things this way [i.e. through compulsory and universal measures] it wouldn't work at all. It changed people's ideas about what was medically possible.[35]

War-time doctors learned this lesson well: that a determined medical service, armed with specific drugs and limitless disciplinary powers, could make a whole army well, no matter what the soldiers thought about it. It was a lesson which would inform the medical strategy of the post-war colonial administration.

The Pacific War marks a decisive break in the history of medical services in colonial Papua New Guinea. From the 1880s until the end of the war, medical administrators attempted to deal with highly specific manifestations of illness, relying on quarantine and quinine, and treating yaws and hookworm in the Melanesian population. Colonialism, and particularly the new forms of social organisation on plantations, mining fields, the little towns and the missions stations, created foci for a wide range of quite new infections, whose tide was too great for the few medical authorities to stem. By the end of the Pacific War, during which many of the pre-war controls and programmes were disrupted, Melanesians were probably fewer, and suffered a wider range of illness, than ever before.[36]

2
The rise and fall of the great campaigns

8
Miracle drugs, new perceptions and the post-war Public Health Department

The Pacific War was slow to wind up in New Guinea. Japanese forces – cut off but still able to defend themselves – were harassed by Australian and Papua New Guinean soldiers, while MacArthur drove on to Manila. It was late in 1945 before all surrenders were accepted, all conscript labourers returned home, and most military detachments demobilised. During six years of war (including almost four of direct combat) many features of the 1930s had been obliterated. In particular, the post-war medical administration would be armed with a range of new drugs and animated by new perceptions of medical possibilities. Most obviously, penicillin became available. It was used widely in the armed services but more sparingly among civilians. The first instance of penicillin being used for a civilian's traumas, may have occurred in 1943: a young Milne Bay girl was carried by the missionary Cecil Abel to a military hospital, her arm so badly broken and infected that he thought she would lose it. The medical officer on duty administered penicillin lavishly – Abel was jolted by the unspoken calculation that several hundred pounds' worth of the drug had been administered – and miraculously the girl's arm was saved.[1] Civilian doctors in peace-time were less lavish in prescribing it, at the price which it commanded, but gradually it became cheaper and more accessible.

Equally arresting was the power of sulpha drugs. Strictly speaking, these existed before the war, and there is at least one instance of their being used in the Solomon Islands during the late 1930s.[2] War accelerated the production and distribution of sulphaguanadine, which (to cite an extreme instance) was supplied generously during the war-time epidemic of dysentery in the New Guinea highlands.[3] Dr John Gunther, a doctor in the backwaters of the Solomon Islands and north Queensland until the war swept him into the Royal Australian Air Force and the New Guinea Campaign, remembered administering up to 27 pills in a single dose.[4] Meanwhile, in a most astonishing piece of individual research inspiration, streptomycin was being isolated as a reliable cure for tuberculosis.[5]

Until the Pacific War, most sick people anywhere, who could be treated at all, would regain their health through the work of nurses. The miracle drugs changed that: sick people would now be drugged back to health rather than nursed. The further consequence was to change the nature of nursing, gradually transforming a relatively independent profession into an ancillary one, in which the nurse's prime function was to supervise the recovery of patients who were responding to drugs prescribed by doctors. General practice would also be transformed, as treatment became standardised.

So long as most infections were either incurable, or at best required long and intensive nursing, it was medically wise to segregate (or to quarantine) the sick from the healthy, and to separate the chronically sick – or even the potentially sick – from their healthy peers. The whole basis of the quarantine strategy (which Cilento articulated so clearly)[6] was to isolate healthy individuals from potential infection. The impact of the miracle drugs on medical thinking was therefore profound, even if the implementation of new programmes was somewhat slower: infections which were now curable (or more easily cured) no longer posed quite the same threat, and no longer justified such strict control over human movement. Quarantine regulations persisted, but they lost their earlier salience.

In any event, a quarantine strategy was becoming logistically impossible. War set tens of thousands of men and women in motion across the face of the earth; in peace-time the scale and speed of human movement hardly slackened, as road and air transport became more common. The consequence for public health policy was to add urgency to programmes which would treat the whole population, rather than segments of it. If it was impractical to exclude any infections, then the whole population should be fore-armed to resist or to survive it.

Implicit in that view of the world was the assumption that medical programmes could not rely upon voluntary cooperation. Army doctors had vivid experience of imposing health upon whole armies through unquestioning discipline: what worked for armies would surely work for civilians. Nor were national borders any longer significant in quite the old way. The World Health Organisation, created at the end of the war, provided machinery to coordinate every medical service on the planet.

Pre-war medical policies had often assumed that most prevailing infections were endemic, and that only a minority of sufferers could be cured. Post-war medical policies often reflected the belief that specific forms of infection were avoidable. This change in outlook was reflected in campaigns to eliminate sleeping sickness from tropical Africa, yellow fever internationally, and malaria in several parts of the Mediterranean. Malaria eradication involved campaigns to eliminate anopheles mosquitoes, through the massive application of DDT. Robert Black characterises such afflictions as follows:

> they are infections which a central health authority, equipped with an adequate supply of drugs or insecticides and a small staff can attack in a way which requires a minimum of cooperation from the community.[7]

By the time Black delivered this lecture (1958) he recognised that public health programmes of this kind were incompatible with a fully democratic political system. But Papua New Guinea at the end of the war was in no sense a democratic society.

These universal shifts in perception were matched in Australia by a quite new range of possibilities in the field of colonial administration and development. The Australian administrations between the wars had not seized every public health opportunity which presented itself: the post-war administration would be more vigorous than before, in consequence of significant changes in Australian government itself.

The Australian federal capital, Canberra, manifested the resources which the federating states made available to the Commonwealth. Although a (temporary) parliament house opened its doors in the 1920s, there was little other evidence of a government. The small revenue base of the Commonwealth did not allow much of a bureaucracy. Many departments remained physically in Melbourne until the 1940s. That fraction of the bureaucracy which took up residence in Canberra formed a tiny community perched on the edge of the older and more substantial country town of Queanbeyan in New South Wales. The office which dealt with external territories comprised a handful of men, shunted from major department to department. That office was too small to initiate policy: most of its work was replying to letters of complaint. When war broke out, and civilian administration was suspended in New Guinea and Papua, the Department of Defence assumed bureaucratic responsibility for the duration, directing ANGAU as a quasi-civilian administration of occupied territory, and employing a research directorate to contemplate post-war reconstruction.[8]

The fact of war persuaded the federated states to surrender extensive powers to the Commonwealth. Those powers – notably the power to levy income tax – remained with the Commonwealth in peace time, entrenching the federal government on the commanding height of the national economy, dispensing largesse to the states – and to the Territory of Papua New Guinea – on an unprecedented scale.[9] Just as Canberra out-grew neighbouring Queanbeyan and eventually incorporated it as a de facto suburb, so Port Moresby (the administrative headquarters of the combined administration of Papua and New Guinea, from 1946) out-grew Hanuabada, and incorporated it as an urban village. Here, at last, was an administration with real resources.

But to what purpose? When the Department of Territories resumed responsibility for Papua and New Guinea, its officers could identify no basis for a colonial economy. Mineral production dwindled; plantations recovered only slowly from war-destruction; manufacturing lacked human and physical infrastructure. Some kind of economic activity seemed appropriate, in order to strengthen Papua New Guinea as a shield against invasion[10] – but what kind of activity was feasible? The Department was advised that

> since Australia's security is paramount, if in order to develop the country and keep it developed it is necessary to subsidise Europeans so as to cause them to

remain in production, the Government must be prepared to pay these subsidies.[11]

It became embarrassingly clear that 'development' would be a very slow and difficult process, in which the role of the territorial administration should be:

a to locate, assess and regulate the availability of natural resources so as to conserve these resources and so as to bring them within reach for development by private capital wherever possible;
b to regulate the availability of the labour force, i.e.
    i to increase the size of the force, and
    ii to ensure the most economic and efficient use of the force available;
c to attract (not provide) the capital necessary to develop the resources.[12]

The centrality of public health programmes was underlined by the belief that the existing population (estimated at 1,500,000) could safely yield only a maximum of 90,000 workers, otherwise the fabric of rural society might be destroyed. Since coloured immigration was unthinkable, and white immigration wildly unlikely, the only way to increase the labour force was to increase the indigenous population, and to make it more productive. The mechanism for generating this increased and more efficient labour force was 'improvements in Health, Education, and the general standard of living, and, perhaps more important of all, through the preservation of the family unit'.

Much of this policy discussion was fanciful. However, this approach would encourage any medical plan which held out hope of a larger or healthier population. The new vision of medical planners would generate many proposals which satisfied the new criteria, and would unlock the new funds available to the Commonwealth.

The most urgent task in re-building a public health programme was to appoint a Director of Public Health. The Commonwealth Director-General of Health appealed to the Repatriation Commission for the release of Dr Bruce Sinclair:

> The External Territories Department is anxious to make a good show of their resumption of [civilian] control and Sinclair is their remaining senior officer of the old Service.[13]

Some senior officers had been killed, and others diverted to new positions. Seventeen men applied, and six were short-listed. Ranked second by the Director-General was Dr John Gunther:

> Dr Gunther is strongly recommended by the RAAF authorities as a suitable appointee. He has a good war record in the Territory [including a successful research project into scrub typhus], and pre-war experience in the Solomons [working for Lever Brothers]. It is considered that Dr B. A. Sinclair has the qualifications and experience and personal qualities which make him the first selection. He is aged 49, while Dr Gunther is 35.[14]

Sinclair could not be released, and the Department of Territories took the plunge, appointing an exceptionally young man to an unusually demanding position. He shared some of the qualities of Colonel Honman a generation earlier – hard-crusted, soft-hearted, not frightened of alcohol or anything else. He had, however, mastered the skills which the job required. Jinks describes him in these terms:

> Gunther possessed a most forceful personality, which he could use to dramatise his own demands, and in all his work he accomplished something rare in Papua New Guinea: setting clear objectives and working, with sometimes ruthless dedication, towards them. At a time when many of the plans for Papua New Guinea were unformed, this ability in the Director was to prove of enormous benefit to the public health effort, although it sometimes meant that other projects went short of scarce materials when their proponents were unable to withstand Gunther's demands. Gunther could be blunt to the point of rudeness and never hesitated to voice his opinions, which were both liberal, for the time, and pragmatic: he believed that achieving results was the best way of supporting a principle.[15]

On his first visit to Port Moresby, on a tour of inspection, he rivetted the attention of the Administrator and the Government Secretary – who kept him waiting for appointments – by telling them to get stuffed.[16] He was not kept waiting again.

The proposed appointment of Sinclair attested to the Department of Territories' preference for experience. Gunther was willing to learn from his elders, but he consulted them in vain. A handful of pre-war doctors and medical assistants returned to the civilian administration, but they had no administrative experience, and were not brought into policy-making positions.[17] Walter Mersh Strong was senile, and unable to explain how he had run Papuan services. Instead, he needed a male orderly to look after him. Eric Wright, formerly a medical assistant and now qualified as a doctor, struck Gunther as an unreliable informant.[18] Sir Raphael Cilento was busy campaigning to be head of the World Health Organisation; Tom Brennan was supportive, but preoccupied with repatriation work.[19] Willy-nilly, it was not pre-war but war-time experience which was the shared background of most medical personnel in Papua New Guinea and in most of the world – rapid transport, a certain brusqueness in style, and enthusiasm for the miracle drugs to combat the killing diseases. These were the main sources of the new department's values and procedures, and the inspiration of its campaigns.

The heads of other departments muttered about Gunther hogging the territorial budget. In practice, his department never received more than the proportion which the New Guinea department had enjoyed in the 1930s.[20] It was only because the budget itself was infinitely more generous than before, that Public Health enjoyed improved funding. It is possible to compare the major allocations in the new administration between 1946 and 1949: see table 3.[21]

The figures explain the irritation of the other departmental heads.

Table 3

Department	1946–7	1947–8	1948–9
District services and native affairs	£368,540	£536,790	£638,236
Public health	173,191	326,063	605,735
Education	36,695	103,008	147,237
Agriculture, stock & fish	46,798	91,567	190,916

Gunther was certainly a talented mobilizer of resources. From the departing Australian and American forces, he scrounged material which they would have bulldozed into the ground – the camaraderie of doctors ensured that departing medical officers preferred to see their material used rather than destroyed.[22] Again, there was an acute shortage of housing, and the Commonwealth Department of Works responded faster to demands in Australia itself, than for houses and hospitals in remote Papua New Guinea. In the short run, Gunther was the most ruthless of the departmental heads commandeering empty buildings; and in the long run he had the management and political skills to present an overwhelming case for hospital construction.[23] By 1950 he could report a total of 51 hospitals sprinkled throughout the country, compared with 21 in 1940 (though his statistics were, characteristically, dubious).[24] Accommodation could be 'stretched' as some medical assistants built their own, and by insisting that medical officers be single (de facto if not de jure) and share whatever accommodation did exist.[25]

A more serious constraint was the shortage of medical staff. Doctors were in short supply, in Australia as much as anywhere else. In 1950 Gunther reckoned that he had only a dozen doctors treating patients, apart from those who were resigning, on leave, or (as in his own case) administering the department. On that calculation, he deployed fewer doctors than his predecessors.[26] In those circumstances, every doctor was a general practitioner, and nobody specialised.[27] On the other hand, the end of the war released large numbers of dressers or ward orderlies, whose skills were better appreciated in Papua New Guinea than in peace-time Australia. European medical assistants responded to advertisements offering a salary of £710 to £734 per annum, and requiring: 'Trained male nurse of experience in tropical disease pattern of native people preferred. Minimum requirements are St. John's Ambulance Certificate in First Aid and/or Home Nursing Certificate, or equivalent.'

The duties were 'under supervision to assist in the conduct of native hospitals; also native hygiene; medical records, stores and ration issues'.[28] When civilian administration resumed at the end of 1945, the provisional government deployed 52 medical assistants. Gunther demanded at least twice that number, and began to search for the pre-war Assistants. Eighteen of them were back in harness (or returning to duty) in February 1946; six were not interested; and nine had yet to decide. A year later, 25 of the pre-war assistants had been tempted back into service, in a complement of 61.[29] The most senior and experienced medical assistants performed virtually all the functions of a doctor, and earned the pre-war nickname 'liklik dokta'. By 1951 there were 85 of them, and Gunther was still searching for more, to make up his complement of 106 positions.[30] With 85, he was better served than his predecessors; but there were severe limits to the use which could be made of the tough ex-servicemen. Appointed at Grade I, they were not competent to run a bush-materials hospital without supervision until they qualified for promotion to Grades II or III.[31] In particular, the new drugs with their miraculous properties implied a cadre of doctors who had been taught how to use them. In the absence of a large number of doctors, Gunther was obliged very largely to carry through the pre-war programmes, no doubt more thoroughly than his predecessors, but still not the new programmes of eradication and prevention which had become technically possible. A more significant departure from the pre-war practices of public health was the recruitment of nearly 40 female nurses.

Gunther was frustrated. He was young, and impatient, and suffering outraged him as much as sin might offend a missionary: he knew that much suffering was avoidable, if only there were specialist doctors to supervise campaigns against specific killing diseases.[32] His view of medicine was in some ways very conventional: there had to be hospitals, and doctors, and an energetic research programme to service both. Without the supervision which only trained doctors could provide, the European medical assistants were insufficient. As fast as he scoured the countryside by aeroplane and truck and motorcycle, what he mainly discovered was avoidable suffering. With all his ruthless, administratively inspired, and patient-centred efforts, and his ability to inspire his staff to heroic self-exploitation, he had not constructed an adequate medical service by 1950.

Many curious conventions hedged the recruitment of doctors for the Australian territories. An Australian Army Captain applied for appointment. The acting Director-General noted that the applicant (otherwise acceptable) was indisputably Chinese, though married to a non-Chinese Australian. The interview officer reported that 'I do not consider that his Chinese appearance would unduly prejudice people against him as it is offset by his Australian manner and satisfactory personality'.[33] This case did not come to Gunther's notice, but he would probably have complained about it, because he was outraged by two other forms of social discrimination which hampered recruitment. One was the reluctance of the Department of Territories in Canberra to appoint women doctors. The first woman to break the barrier was Dr Joan Refshauge, who was advised by the Secretary of the department to re-train as an obstetrician and gynaecologist, since there could be no question of her treating black men, in sickness or in health.[34] To Gunther this was simply humbug: a doctor was a doctor.[35] (He did not, on the other hand, dispel the equally sexist and racist tradition that white women nurses should tend only white patients.)[36]

The other grievous discrimination was the reluctance of registration boards and the British Medical Association in Australia (now the Australian Medical Association) to recognise the medical qualifications of European doctors, who were present in Australia as displaced persons.[37] They first came to the attention of the territory when Gunther noticed some apparently qualified doctors applying from refugee camps in Australia for employment as medical assistants. In order to employ them as doctors, he had to contend with fierce opposition from Australian ex-servicemen through the Returned Services League, Australian doctors through the British Medical Association, and even the Australian Director-General of Health. And he won: during 1950 he interviewed, recruited, and deployed 50 Hungarians, Poles, Ukrainians and other central Europeans. At one bound, the department quadrupled its establishment of doctors, and was able to pursue many of the campaigns which Gunther had planned. Where the pre-war Health Departments were content to reflect social prejudice, the new department resolutely opposed it.

By 1956, when he ceased to be Director, Gunther had created what may have been one of the finest medical services of that era in a tropical dependency. Its programmes will be considered later: here it is instructive to consider the circumstances which made it possible. First, this was the high noon of Australian colonial administration, untroubled by nationalist resistance or imminent decolonisation. The militarist style, which most doctors and nurses and medical assistants carried over from the war, could express itself fully. It was a criminal offence for anyone to disobey medical instructions.[38] Secondly, the colonial administration had only the vaguest of development strategies, so that almost any convincing case for expenditure was likely to be funded. Gunther believed that his capacity to spend money effectively was unusual among departmental heads: he certainly did not lack that capacity. Thirdly, medical science and doctors were held in higher public esteem after the war than ever before. Not only did bureaucrats defer to them, but so did villagers, so that the penal provisions of the criminal code were hardly ever invoked. Finally, the miracle drugs were at their peak of effectiveness in 'virgin field' conditions: with hindsight (but only with hindsight) we know that their victories would prove less conclusive than they seemed.

These circumstances need not have combined to create a good public health service: it was Gunther who turned them to advantage. Sir William Refshauge made this judgment of Gunther's administration:

> In public health it is almost all administration that counts. That is not belittling the field workers at all; but unless you have a good administration, you don't get the field staff moving, and you don't get the material to them. The district clinics and the hospitals don't get built, or equipped. Gunther did an almost impossible job, given the difficulty of communication and transport. He had

some funny people on his staff, and he recruited some funny people too; but at least he produced people who were doing things. He was also producing facilities which were better than they had ever had.[39]

Stan Christian served as a medical assistant to every Director from Cilento to Scragg, but Gunther was the first he ever met face to face. Gunther would visit him in the Wahgi valley, to see for himself how the malaria-control experiments were developing, then tear off on a motor-cycle into a cloud of dust.[40] Gunther was not only a capable scrounger and a successful manager of resources but, equally importantly, he was a brilliant inspirer of his staff. His department was wildly polyglot, men and women, black and white, ocker and reffo: Gunther welded them into a service which commanded, and received, remarkable respect.

Gunther was a passionate patriot, convinced of the special ability of Australians to discharge their medical trust towards Papua New Guineans. His confidence in his staff of new Australians, and in the old Australian scientists who moved from the army to research positions in Australia, made him skeptical of international organisations. He kept the South Pacific Commission at arm's length, and his enthusiasm for the World Health Organisation was tempered by its policy of not sending Australian specialists to the Australian dependency.[41] In the mid-1950s he made every effort to exclude the American researcher Carleton Gajdusek from the *kuru* investigation: *kuru* was peculiar to the Australian territory, and therefore a subject which Australian scientists were obliged (and he believed able) to unravel.[42]

Yet Australian public health institutions offered no model to emulate. Since the Great War, the Commonwealth Government had acknowledged a responsibility towards ex-service men and women, and provided them with admirable health facilities through the Repatriation Department. The rest of the civilian population were not so lucky: even when the British Government enacted the National Health Service, the Australian Government was content to leave most civilian medical services in private hands. Neither of these parallel structures was relevant to the Papua New Guinea case: in order to discharge Australia's responsibility, Gunther was bound to turn his back on Australian precedent as well as his New Guinean and Papuan predecessors. There was never the slightest question that Papua New Guineans individually – nor even the territory as a whole – should shoulder the financial burden of effective public health.

A later generation of commentators would compare the new Public Health Department with the 'barefoot doctors' of the People's Republic of China.[43] That analogy was also well wide of the mark. What the new department attempted was the fullest possible application of *western* medical procedures, through the conventional personnel of doctors and nurses and health extension officers, with complete disregard to financial realism. The department became the centrepiece of a welfare colonialism which bore little resemblance to possible precedents, and which was thoroughly empirical in seeking out the best available methods, judged only by professional criteria. In a colonial administration staffed by technicists, the Department of Health was unusual only in its élan and its effectiveness.

9
The health campaigns

Although most of the personnel were new, and conscious of making a new beginning in public health, in one respect at least they persisted in old habits. Most of the activity of the department was correctly described as a series of assaults on specific diseases. The purpose of Gunther's survey of before he assumed the Directorship, was to identify the 'killer-diseases' which posed the most serious threats to health, and which were most amenable to treatment. His exasperation during the first years of his office was the shortage of personnel to attack the diseases which he had targeted. In retrospect this may seem to have been a strategic error; but the approach was shared by public health authorities throughout the world, and war-time habits of thought easily seduced medical workers to see specific disease as the enemy. During the 1950s that mind-set was, if anything, reinforced. Counter-insurgency campaigns during the 1950s often endorsed the medical image of communism and nationalist revolt as unnatural infections to be contained and eradicated by heroic effort. To be sure, the excitement of campaigning against specific diseases did wonders for the morale of ex-servicemen doctors, and evoked heroism in their work. Perhaps no other strategy could have been so readily understood by the medical workers, nor so enthusiastically implemented.

Malaria became the prime target. The assault was inspired more by the increasing self-confidence of doctors, than by new chemotherapy. The first phase of the campaign, in fact, involved little more than the resolute application of old techniques which had been neglected throughout the 1930s. Gunther's recollection was that

> all of us who worked in Melanesia before the war knew that, with a little effort, we could do more than we were doing, against malaria. We could distribute gambusia fish [which fed on mosquito spawn]; we could have introduced quinine to the village people; but it was said that giving quinine would upset their natural immunity. It was these views that were altered in war time. We found that, by discipline, we could keep whole armies free of malaria. We knew that, by engineering methods, we could reduce the mosquito population. We knew that, with drugs, we could suppress malaria in the native population, without interfering greatly with their immunity.[1]

New regulations required employers to dose their workers with suppressives; and the inception of the Highlands Labour Scheme in 1949 – which brought non-immune highlanders to coastal regions of hyper-endemic malaria – added urgency to this regulation. Even then, Gunther relied on his personal friendships with planters, to have the regime imposed. On one appalling occasion he had a plantation manager dismissed for disregarding regulations – after enjoying the man's hospitality the night before the inspection.[2]

The model which inspired the programme was not merely the realisation of pre-war opportunities lost, but the eradication of malaria from Sardinia immediately after the Second World War.[3] However, if the original dream was complete eradication (through the interruption of transmission rather than the elimination of anopheles mosquitoes entirely), it soon became a campaign to establish *control*. An early pilot project, which involved residual spraying of DDT, yielded discouraging results. The actual behaviour of anopheles mosquitoes was not yet well enough understood; and the pilot project did not run long enough to give conclusive evidence.[4] Not until the mid-1950s was a more comprehensive campaign launched. It was supported by detailed research on water tables and their control, and on mosquito behaviour in a variety of environments, to determine where and when they were most vulnerable. The cutting edges of the campaign were residual spraying of houses with DDT, and of bodies of stagnant water which were too extensive to be drained.[5]

Because malaria weakened people's resistance to other infections, and had such a diffuse and debilitating effect on whole populations, Gunther stuck to his campaign. When he marshalled all his arguments, they were almost irresistible:

> Control malaria and double the expectation of life;
> Control malaria and halve the infant mortality rate;
> Control malaria and double the population in fifteen to twenty years;
> Control malaria and add 15% to the efficiency of the individual labourer;
> Control malaria and reduce the potential need for labour by 25%;
> Control malaria and therefore save hundreds of thousands of pounds;
> And, of great significance, Control malaria and improve the aptitude of the pupil or the student by up to 25%[6]

Results never quite matched the rhetoric. Control over water tables, and the resolute spraying of all houses and stagnant water courses, required a degree of popular and bureaucratic cooperation which could not be achieved, let alone sustained. In 1957 two full-scale pilot projects were initiated:

> Although transmission of malaria was not interrupted, the results achieved demonstrated that malaria control using residual spraying would be of considerable benefit to the country. The results also showed that, with a concerted effort and a high degree of administrative support and public cooperation, interruption of transmission was highly probable.[7]

Even in the circumscribed areas of the pilot programmes, success was uncertain and conditional. During the 1960s the programme was extended to cover about half of the countryside; but as it expanded it met increasing resistance:

> The programme by this time was hampered by its unpopularity with the people, both in the rural situation and Administration and private sectors. Open antagonism was often the case. Expansion was stopped in 1969 and a period of stabilization and sorting was undertaken.[8]

Once the expansion was halted, it was not resumed.

No single reason accounts for the halting of the campaign. Rather, it exemplified the common life cycle of any organised medical programme against a specific infection, beginning with delight in new possibilities, running to despair as technical and social problems mounted, and to the need to re-think the problem. As Charlwood sadly observes, a complex epidemiology such as malaria can quite readily cope with even ruthless control measures. The initial impact of DDT was exceptional – but not repeatable.[9] Furthermore, malaria was expanding faster than it was being controlled. The building of roads into the highlands, and the entry of infected outsiders (and returning highland migrants) brought malaria to previously inaccessible regions. The least accessible part of the highlands is Enga province. By the end of the 1970s, malaria had become endemic in the Sau river valley at altitudes ranging from 800 to 1800 metres, bringing anaemia and stunted growth. Even the Lagaip River Valley – between 1800 and 2400 metres – had occasional cases of malaria.[10] Between the increasing objections of the people to residual spraying, the declining effectiveness of control measures, and the manifest expansion of malaria beyond its earlier boundaries, the campaign gradually became mired. A measure of the problem is the revival, in the 1970s and 1980s, of appeals for village-based health education and community-based efforts to make life difficult for the anopheles mosquito.[11]

If malaria was the prime target, then tuberculosis was certainly the second. Little was done about the distribution of the tubercle bacillus until the 1940s. Europeans and Polynesians who came to live in the territories included infectious victims of the 'white plague', and medical officers reported gloomily on its seemingly inevitable advance.[12] Only in the 1930s, when Dr Heydon found tuberculosis almost entirely absent from the highlands, did the question become salient in the minds of medical planners. The bacillus was most common in Hanuabada, the peri-urban Papuan village being incorporated into Port Moresby: tuberculosis was clearly a consequence of exposure to colonialism.[13] The initiative had been taken by those villagers who were its chief victims: one Hanuabadan decided to contribute to the communal good by building an isolation hospital. With the support and encouragement of the London Missionary Society, the villagers set Gemo Island apart as an isolation hospital for tuberculosis and leprosy. In the conditions of the 1930s, that was the most that could be done. Even that was not done very well: advanced cases were sometimes sent home to die, perhaps through an injudicious sympathy with the particular victim. And the outbreak of the Pacific War, which led to the closing of all isolation hospitals, distributed all the known cases back to their homes.[14]

Until the 1940s, the most effective measure available was vaccination with Bacille Calmette-Guerin (BCG), which could drastically reduce the incidence of the disease in a given population, but did not provide complete immunity. Prospects improved dramatically during the 1940s, when Dr Selman Waksman isolated streptomycin, and controlled trials proved it to be the basis for successful treatment.[15] Tuberculosis was now both avoidable and treatable, and John Gunther planned a campaign as soon as he had sufficient staff to encompass it. Dr Edgar North of the Commonwealth Serum Laboratory was invited to Papua New Guinea in 1949 to discuss the use of BCG and towards the end of 1950 Gunther formally proposed a 'Programme to Control Tuberculosis'.[16] The programme would involve mass vaccination with BCG; concentrating on the highlands region and its vulnerable and susceptible population; and it hinged upon the Commonwealth Serum Laboratory's ability to supply freeze-dried vaccine (instead of the usual wet vaccine) in order to bring BCG to those parts of the country where transport was slow and unreliable. The project included provision for surgical units in many of the hospitals, where a visiting team of surgeons could perform remedial surgery; but the campaign was mainly a preventive one, and Gunther made it clear that prevention had a higher priority than the long-term need for hospitals and surgical units.

The proposal flew in the face of established procedures. It relied on the new, freeze-dried vaccine, and it gave priority to the nearly-virgin population rather than the communities where tuberculosis was already entrenched. Dr Harry Wunderly of the Division of Tuberculosis in the Commonwealth Department of Health queried the strategy late in 1951, and asked why thoracic surgery facilities were needed in so many different hospitals.[17] Gunther overcame these objections, and the campaign swung into operation early in the 1950s.

An active research programme proceeded concurrently with the BCG vaccinations. Australian scientists were heavily involved, and in the countryside the missions gave enthusiastic support, providing the isolation hospitals for long-term care. The Tuberculosis Unit worked autonomously, with its own extension workers in the field. The BCG programme was integrated into the Highlands Labour Scheme, which required that all highland recruits be vaccinated. After some unsatisfactory attempts by staff of the TB unit, teams of Australian surgeons were brought in from time to time to operate on victims who were marshalled for their visits. During the decade ending in 1966, over 700 operations were performed. This procedure had been abandoned in Australia early in the 1950s, and there must be some question about its usefulness in Papua New Guinea, but it was an impressive feat of organisation to have them done at all. The programme operated far beyond the economic capacity of the country. As Wigley delicately put it:

> the cost of the programme, although determined basically by Departmental priorities, was considered solely in the light of the obligation of ... Australia to overcome the problem as quickly as possible, rather than by any considerations of a developing country's capacity to support the cost.[18]

In one sense, this commitment and obligation was only fair. There may have been no tuberculosis in the country at all, before colonialism; and its progress through the population almost exactly replicated exposure to the colonial economy. By 1970, for example, exposure to infection ranged from 66 per cent in Port Moresby down to 7 per cent in isolated Lumi. It was still rare in children under fifteen years of age; and among adults it was five times as common among males as among females.[19] The inexorable bond between 'development' and 'disease' lent urgency to this programme, while the prospect was still available of protecting large numbers of people before they were exposed. And the campaign was very successful. The peak number of patients in hospital or domiciliary care was 5,000 in 1964–65; by 1970 the case load had steadied at about 3,000 and fewer than 2,000 cases per annum were being detected. By that time, tuberculosis was no longer a national crisis, but a relatively minor public health problem.[20] If the campaign (like the malaria campaign) passed through a climax of excitement and high morale, it did not sink to quite the same depths of despair.

A third apparently avoidable disease which disfigured post-war Papua New Guinea was leprosy. Isolation had been the leading strategy until the war. When Dr Joan Refshauge assumed responsibility for Gemo Island isolation settlement (as part of her Port Moresby duties), she found that the LMS had re-assembled lepers after their war-time dispersal. She also discovered – as diagnostic measures became more sensitive, and visiting specialists more common – that some of her patients had been incorrectly diagnosed.[21] The new programme also stressed the discovery and isolation of sufferers, and their long-term treatment. As the mission medical services were better equipped than the Department to offer long-term care, the programme was largely delegated to them.[22] The problem surrounding leprosy treatment was not so much the care of patients, as their discovery. By 1970, some 15,000 cases had been diagnosed, but Russell and Bell estimated that about half as many cases continued to elude the medical patrols.[23]

In 1983 Dr S. G. Browne remarked that

> clinical impressions gained over wide areas of newly-diagnosed patients suffering from preventible deformities which had not been prevented, or from signs of advancing lepromatous disease, suggest that all is not well.

Brown identified the long-standing problems of failed diagnosis, and poor cooperation by patients in long-term treatment, and he added the newly discovered hazards of dapsone-resistant strains of leprosy, and the ability of the causative organism to remain dormant for months or years.[24] Leprosy, like so many other infections, had survived an organised campaign and discovered means of flourishing in a slightly changed environment.

There were other campaigns, of varying intensity, depending partly upon the expertise which Gunther and his successor (Dr Roy Scragg) had available. They ranged from short-term crisis infections such as pneumonia and diarrhoea, through to persistent problems such as sexually transmitted diseases; and from the dramatic such as polio and *kuru* to the commonplace yaws. It is not the intention of this study to describe all the campaigns, still less to evaluate them, but to suggest some of their more significant features.

The characteristic feature of these campaigns was best described by Robert Black in 1958, in a passage already quoted:

> The feature common to all these diseases where success has been achieved and which is largely responsible for this success is: they are infections which a central health authority, equipped with an adequate supply of drugs or insecticides and a small staff can attack in a way which requires a minimum of cooperation from the community. There is little or no local effort, no local understanding required. Thus malaria is dealt with by teams spraying the walls of houses with DDT, yaws by teams giving a single injection of penicillin.[25]

A consequence of this central organisation was to create profound dependence upon the central authority: if the campaign broke down, nothing that a village community could do would sustain it.[26] Especially through the 1960s, when colonialism itself was yielding to local democratic participation, popular resentment emerged against the intrusiveness of the campaign workers. For Black, the proper solution was to develop health education as the campaigns reached their technical limits. The recommendation was logical, but it was also impractical, given the number of languages spoken in the countryside, the shortage of trained health extension officers, the technicist values of the doctors, and the diversity of environmental and epidemiological circumstances.

A second feature of the campaign approach to public health was a certain ad hoc quality. Gunther recollected the drafting of many health plans, none of which he intended as a guide to action.[27] As expertise cropped up – in tuberculosis, or leprosy, or child health – so campaigns were built around the personnel. Each campaign had its own headquarters staff and research facility, its own regional direction, and its own field officers; and as the campaigns proliferated, so the task of coordination in each district became more daunting.[28] While Gunther could animate his staff, and personally coordinate supplies and staff, he could contain the contradictions between segmented campaign direction and pyramidal public health administration; but this was not a long-term solution.

One of the penalties of a campaign-based department, which relied on

Canberra ultimately for its funding, was to become over-committed to the struggle with specific infections. The dramatic quality of a disease, a necessary condition for raising funds to control it, implied an autonomous unit to tackle it. Yet each unit, with its shared skills, added to the difficulty of national coordination.

Opportunities seized were matched by opportunities foregone. During 1947 a most impressive and comprehensive New Guinea Nutrition Survey was conducted, at the request of the Department of Territories.[29] The survey was an exemplary combination of scientific skills: biochemists, parasitologists, nutritionists, agronomists, anthropologists and dentists pooled their perceptions. The territorial departments of Health, Education, Agriculture, and District Services were involved in the planning. Five villages were selected for intensive investigation, reflecting the environmental diversity. The report was published, with lavish illustrations. And it was never again referred to. The survey created a baseline for precisely the kinds of integrated health programmes which would be acceptable in the 1970s, but which could not be carried out in the 1950s. So obsessed were medical officers with the particular campaigns which they were waging, that there was simply no scope for what would later be called 'community medicine'.

This predicament was not simply the product of Gunther's adhocracy: it arose directly out of the perceived health hazards of the era. The air-fields and roads which allowed medical personnel their new access to remote areas were at the same time the arteries of infection. There was a real race between the pathology and the therapy of development, and it was the excitement of this race which animated the health workers of the new department. In these dramatic circumstances, the department could hardly have performed differently – and perhaps no department could have performed better. Yet Robert Black was profoundly right in his analysis of the centrally directed campaigns. The miracle drugs yielded decreasing returns; an uninformed public became increasingly resistant to arbitrary direction; and the glorious set piece warfare of the first years of each campaign led on to the frustrations and immobilism of guerilla warfare. Trained and inspired for the formal campaigns, the department was temperamentally unsuited to battles which could have no triumphant conclusion.

Medical workers were possessed by a sense of failure in the later 1960s, as each field campaign ran into unexpected technical and social obstacles. Considered less emotionally, however, the era of specific disease campaigns is not a disaster. During a generation of expansion, the scale of the department had increased; the earlier focus on enclaves of expatriates and wage labourers was replaced by a genuine enthusiasm for the health of the whole rural population; the research which accompanied each of the campaigns added up to an immense array of precise information; and despair in particular campaigns was the reflection of a continuing determination to bring health to everyone, by more careful attention to the problems which presented themselves. If many diseases had learned how to survive medical assault, the medical workers were also passing through a learning curve which left them less naive and more sophisticated in their appreciation of the public health field. It is no coincidence that standards of health and life expectancy began to improve most sharply, precisely when the great campaigns became exhausted. What was needed was a new strategy to take advantage of accumulated knowledge and persistent commitment.

10
Women and children last

Much of the history of medical administration in Papua New Guinea may be read as the local application of universally agreed prescriptions. In one major area of therapy, however, there was variation within the country. At the risk of over-stating the contrast, it is convenient to present the work of the post-war medical missions as complementary to the department's work.

The department was, of course, responsible for the whole country, and the careers of doctors, nurses, and medical assistants (but not aid post orderlies) took them from one district to another, from rural extension work to headquarters administration or to research duties. Though the hospitals and health centres were fixed, the personnel were highly mobile. Each mission, on the other hand, ministered to a circumscribed area, and careers involved long periods in a single language community. Immobility (often intensified by isolation from other expatriates) encouraged familiarity with the language and society of the neighbourhood. Mission personnel who wished to specialise, commonly transferred to the department. Other kinds of specialisation – for instance Ed Tscharke's study of yaws – might entrench a mission worker ever more deeply in one locality. Tscharke built his own hospital on Karkar island, and ran it for thirty years, specialising in yaws treatment.[1]

In the immediate aftermath of war, the missions were financially straitened: their personnel accepted lower salaries than their departmental counterparts, and they managed without expensive technology. Their capacity to absorb high technology was in any case limited by reliance on their own electric power generators. In the course of time, several missions did build well-equipped hospitals (such as the Lutheran hospital at Yagaun outside Madang), more commonly in rural settings than in district headquarters. Even then the prevailing mood was rustic. To some extent the department encouraged the rustication of medical missions. Gunther advised a meeting of medical missionaries in 1946, that

> missionaries, as individuals, are more suited to conduct certain ancillary medical establishments, such as Infant and Maternal Welfare Centres, Leprosaria, and the Institutions for the care of the Tuberculous.[2]

Whereas the department relied upon base-hospitals to which difficult cases should be referred by the localities, each mission service was relatively self-contained: not only the staff, but also the patients, were less mobile than their government counterparts.

There was a less sharp, but still discernible contrast between the dominance of male doctors within the department (except in Maternal and Child Health, which absorbed most of the government's female doctors) and the missions in which women were better represented in positions of authority. Mission nurses, too, were more likely to be female than were the department's nurses. They exercised wide authority, since the proportion of doctors seems to have been relatively low in the missions. To over-state matters, the department was highly mobile, technical, and masculine, catering predominantly to urban and mobile patients: and the missions were immobile, technically simple, relatively feminine, more adept at nursing than at doctoring, catering mainly to rural and immobile patients.

These circumstances alone meant that more women and children were cared for by the missions, than by the department. And the missions liked it that way. Christian medical services are especially committed to 'suffer the little children'.[3] Many of their staff were fluent in the vernaculars, and long enough resident to enjoy the confidence of the mothers of those children. Between the wars, the missions had virtually monopolised maternal and child services for Papua New Guineans: that tradition persisted with few modifications. What was new was the massive commitment of the Administration to organising maternal and child care.

The significance of this programme was clear to the Administrator, Colonel J. K. Murray, a Catholic and a family man. Reporting to his minister in 1949, he developed a most interesting argument:

> The Maternal and Infant Welfare side needs to be given increased attention, not only because of the usual humanitarian considerations, but because the increase in the native population in the Territory is almost certainly a condition of survival ... and is a condition of security as far as this Territory acting as a buffer for Australia is concerned. Many more women medical practitioners are required in order that contact with the native women shall be fully welcomed and effective.[4]

Soon afterwards, in a letter to Senator Kendall, he proposed that there were three methods of resolving the labour shortage: mechanisation of production, highlands labour for coastal plantations, and 'full development of Public Health measures whereby infant and maternal mortality is greatly reduced'. Infant mortality rates, he thought, were often 200, and sometimes 500 per thousand (compared with the Australian rate of 30):

> If we can cut down this appalling loss of child life, there should be a great increase in the native population and the result, in terms of the availability of native labour, apparent within a generation.[5]

These observations clarify several features of the maternal and child health (MCH) service which was taking shape as Murray wrote. The economic and strategic need for increased population is clear enough: and so is the peripheral nature of *maternal* mortality, which was not stated as a problem in itself, but as a dimension of the infant mortality issue. Equally intriguing is Murray's perception of women doctors, no longer anomalous but a positive force for development precisely because of their gender.

The first specialist in maternal and child health was Dr Joan Refshauge. Born into a Victorian family which valued education above everything else, she became a Master of Science and a lecturer in chemistry in Melbourne during the 1930s. When she began to study medicine, she had no particular interest in obstetrics and gynaecology. (Her brother William qualified as a gynaecologist, but the war diverted him to medical administration.) After the war, when Joan wished to join her husband in Papua New Guinea, she was advised to take up the discipline which her brother had abandoned. Many years later, when she was preparing a speech on the subject of sexual discrimination, she reflected:

> I must say discrimination against women was not an issue in my heyday, but on looking back and writing this out I began to realise that there was discrimination, but it was accepted as a fact of life.[6]

She was interviewed by Halligan, the Secretary of the Department of Territories:

> he told me I would be welcome for they were considering starting infant and maternal care, and that was the only work I could do – 'because the Territory was a Man's Country, and men expected men to look after them'. I could never work in a native hospital except if (as was unlikely) babies or mothers were patients. To attend a male patient would endanger other European women. With this understand I did all the right things.

The right things included re-training in obstetrics and gynaecology. Even then there was a delay, because some official reckoned that the appointment of a woman doctor 'would lower the standard of medicine'.[7]

Dr Refshauge arrived before the large infusion of European doctors, and worked as a general practitioner until Gunther felt he could spare her to establish MCH. That task began towards the end of 1948, largely coordinating work already resumed by the Catholic mission at Yule Island, and encouraging other missions to revive their pre-war commitments.[8] Gradually the department began to provide its own personnel: a second woman doctor who was one of the refugee intake of 1950, and several trained female nurses. By 1953 there was an establishment of two doctors, six white sisters, one Papuan assistant mid-wife, and 31 trainees – all female.[9] On out-stations at Kieta, Aitape and Kandrian, clinics were conducted by the wives of European medical assistants and other administration personnel.[10] In a sense, therefore, the unit was still an expression of the old need to have women address the 'peculiar problems' of other women, confining women professionals to purely female tasks. That character would colour the evolution of MCH.

Another persistent trend was observed. Dr Refshauge told the annual mission conference in 1954 that her staff 'found that the infant work gradually became accepted while maternal work lagged behind amongst the native people'.[11] That departmental experience was almost certainly shared by the missions. What was established in the early 1950s was a series of services operated by women, ostensibly for women and children, but actually focused on children. The way in which this perception shaped the service may be inferred from Dr Refshauge's report for 1953–4:

> natives are becoming more conscious of the benefits of ante- and post-natal care, and are now asking for their wives to be admitted to hospitals for confinement, and insisting upon their children attending the welfare clinics . . . In Wewak, the native leader [Pita] Simogun M.L.C., sponsored the building of a Native Maternity Hospital by voluntary workers.

Even in the eyes of the all-women MCH division, Papua New Guinean women were invisible, the shadowy dependents of articulate men. When they do break into the prose of the official reports therefore, they slide out again. Evidently women did want maternal health services, and one paragraph (in a typescript of fourteen pages) acknowledges this:

> Native women have shown an increasing tendency to obtain the full benefits by clinics, especially in ante-natal care and advice. The success achieved is shown by the ease with which native mothers attending the clinics breast-feed their babies, and the number of abnormalities which have been detected and corrected by these clinics. It is planned to give additional talks for mothers, especially in relation to baby foods and the care of babies.[12]

Even an observed demand for *maternal* care leads – within the space of two sentences – to a supply of *child* care, within a paragraph headed *Ante-Natal Care.*

The problem was not simply the artifact of report-writing. Sister Elizabeth Burchill, running a small hospital in Maprik in the Sepik, noted that only six deliveries per month occurred within the hospital, but thought that there was an increasing desire among Sepik women to give birth in the hospital:

> An expectant mother who owed her life to timely surgery through a lucky chance meeting with doctor boy Taro, is not likely to forget Maprik Hospital. At full term, she walked from her village with a loaded bilum on her back (with goods to trade) to the 'bung' one Saturday morning and on arriving felt labour pains come on and increase with alarming intensity. Fortunately, Taro happened to be close by at the time and the woman approached him in her predicament.

Taro persuaded her to come to the hospital, where she spent three hours in the operating theatre, lost the baby, but survived. That incident stands out in a narrative overwhelmingly committed to mothering:

> Preconceived ideas of ancient origin, doubtful customs based on tradition combined with stringent economic need, were retarding factors in Admin-

istration efforts to implement a simple standard of mothercraft within the civilizing influences of the Maprik native hospital.[13]

The care which the Queen Elizabeth II Infant, Child and Maternal Health Service provided for infants and children (if not their mothers) was probably very effective. The staff certainly dabbled with the error, common in other parts of the colonial world, of popularising the consumption of western-style and western-produced baby-foods. The out-stations were provided with Nestlé Condensed Milk, Sunshine Milk, Lactogen, Marmite (but curiously in an Australian dependency, no Vegemite) and cod liver oil.[14] From very early, however, the service was aware of the risks attending that strategy. Dr Refshauge reminded the 1954 Mission Conference that 'many believe that Infant and Maternal Welfare is synonymous with milk supply. The requisition of milk is frequently out of all proportion'. Reliance on cows' milk, she pointed out, was recent even in Europe:

> [and] it is the opinion of . . . F. W. Clement, that one of the tragedies of the last fifty years has been the upsetting of the tradition of native peoples, one of which has been the early weaning of native children, the other the introduction of milk by trade, doctors and missionaries.[15]

Apart from preaching against cows' milk, the service took trouble to develop milk-substitutes from non-dairy and non-imported products.[16]

Coverage was uneven, but MCH services quickly reached a large clientele. By 1956 the statistics at least were impressive. On the Papuan side, the department operated five fixed clinics serving 129 villages; mobile units visited 46 other centres regularly. Missions ran a further 46 clinics. 510 Papuan women had their confinement in department hospitals, and 836 in mission hospitals. On the New Guinea side, 12 fixed clinics served 1,010 villages; 173 centres were visited regularly and nearly 6,000 women gave birth in department or mission hospitals.[17] Van de Kaa carries these figures forward to 1966 (see table 4).[18] Two observations arise directly from these figures. One is the much greater emphasis upon child welfare than upon pre-natal care. The other is the continuing importance of mission organisations in delivering MCH services of any kind. That salience has outlasted colonialism itself. Townsend relates the quality of MCH services provided in each province in the 1980s, not to crude levels of 'development' from place to place, but to the presence or absence of church medical extension workers to supplement the staff of the department.[19]

The effects of these services on the demography of the country have been profound. The gross changes in the national population are well known, with a sustained growth since the 1940s.[20] Less obviously, there may have been a slight 'feminisation' of the population. Van de Kaa's examination of the demographic evidence of the 1960s led him to believe that the female population was growing appreciably faster than the male population. He guessed that 'the female population has profited more from the recent mortality decline than the male population and has therefore grown

Table 4

	Pre-natal clinic attendance (thousands)		Child-welfare clinic attendance (thousands)		Number of	
	Department	Mission	Department	Mission	Hospitals	Aid-posts
1948/49	—	—	—	—	106	258
1958/59	9.6	41.1	236.3	282.5	195	1550
1959/60	11.9	46.4	256.2	325.7	205	1693
1960/61	16.3	50.9	317.0	373.7	213	1689
1961/62	19.8	57.9	350.3	418.2	211	1632
1962/63	24.5	63.1	414.5	506.7	195	1897
1963/64	31.5	70.4	464.6	614.4	217	1614
1964/65	31.2	70.2	507.6	889.3	225	1707
1965/66	31.6	104.4	477.5	993.0	236	1730

faster'.[21] That hypothesis raises many more questions. It is difficult to identify any service available to both sexes, which women might have used disproportionately. And if the observed decline in tribal fighting during the 1960s had any effect on population levels, it should have benefitted men at least as much as women. It is just possible that the introduction of even a limited maternal health service had a short-term effect on the sex ratio of the population at large.

Taking a longer view, the demographic gains made by women in the 1960s were an exception to the general trend. Every attempt to estimate gender ratios throughout the twentieth century has suggested a highly masculine population. In 1973 (even after the hiccup of the 1960s), the official estimate was a masculinity ratio of 111.7 males for every 100 females.[22] The census of 1981 yields almost the same proportion.[23] Let us assume for the moment that Papua New Guinean societies have been highly masculine since the nineteenth century: then how is it that massive changes in the quality and quantity of life, following from changes in standards of living and the provision of health care, have not altered the gender proportions? The care of women was in effect delegated to the Division of Maternal and Child Health, and services were delivered predominantly by the missions within that administrative framework. Michael Young gives us the most significant clue. Within the mission services, there has persistently been a child-centred approach to the delivery of services.[24] His case study on Goodenough Island in Milne Bay documents two entrenched patterns. During the 1960s, mission personnel were so attentive to the health status of children that they admitted something like three-quarters of them to hospital in one year for which there are good records. Only the replacement of the expatriate mission nurses by Papuan nurses ended this gross 'over-servicing' of children. But not all children were over-serviced. Parents were (and remain) twice as likely to bring a sick son to the clinic, as a sick daughter.[25]

Now there may be particular circumstances in Goodenough Island which distinguish it from the rest of the country; but the outcome in massive masculinity ratios is manifest from one end of the country to the other, and indeed seems to be characteristic of the whole Melanesian culture area.[26] Within Papua New Guinea the only province in which females outnumber males is the Southern Highlands, the least 'developed' and therefore the most affected by male out-migration in search of wage labour opportunities. Females are predominantly rural, remaining at home while men congregate in towns and in areas of employment. The division of therapeutic labour between Administration and mission (and now between department and church workers) made women the particular responsibility of mission services: but missions were animated by a commitment to children rather than their mothers. The outcome of female invisibility is the most masculine country on the face of the earth, in which males outnumber females in every age cohort, and increasingly with age. Another way of expressing this situation is to describe Papua New Guinea as one of the most 'motherless' societies on earth.

The low proportion of females in the total population cannot be laid simply at the door of the modern medical services, since high masculinity seems to be an ancient and enduring feature of Melanesian societies generally. The most that can be said is that church and state between them neglected the issue. It is also tempting to lay the blame on 'Melanesian culture', until we remind ourselves that Melanesia encompasses a bewildering array of languages, production systems, inheritance patterns, and styles of living. In order to account for such a diffuse and enduring characteristic, it may be helpful to look sideways at another region of high masculinity, in north India. Barbara Miller contrasts north west India with the rest of the sub-continent, and suggests that the Brahminical tradition lent itself to a marked preference for sons (whereas the Dravidian tradition did not). A long tradition of female infanticide, suppressed or discouraged during the days of the British Raj, persists in the form of selective neglect of female children, so that high levels of masculinity persist. She observed a correlation also between dry-land farming (which has little need of female labour), and an imbalance between dowry and bride-price payments, so that it becomes difficult to point to a single 'cause' for the persistence of the whole complex of attitudes.[27] The north west Indian evidence encourages us to suppose that attitudes towards male and female children can outlast the circumstances which gave rise to them, and that these attitudes may be so deeply buried that parents actually discriminate between their children without noticing that they do so.

Paul Greenough's study of the famine in Bengal in 1943–44[28] offers another clue. In ordinary circumstances, Bengalis acknowledged obligations towards all their dependents. During profound famine, however,

Table 5   *Papua New Guinea population by province, 1980 census*

Province	Persons	Males	Females	Male percentage
Western	78,881	40,232	38,649	52.3
Gulf	64,167	32,718	31,449	51.0
Central	117,242	61,157	56,085	52.2
National Capital	122,761	70,691	52,070	57.6
Milne Bay	127,841	66,832	61,009	52.3
Northern	77,273	41,248	36,025	53.4
Southern Highlands	235,647	115,234	120,413	48.9
Enga	164,476	85,161	79,315	51.8
Western Highlands	262,886	139,689	123,197	53.1
Chimbu	178,490	94,732	83,758	53.1
Eastern Highlands	277,180	143,239	133,941	51.7
Morobe	310,526	159,868	150,658	51.5
Madang	211,209	109,897	101,312	52.0
East Sepik	220,903	111,684	109,219	50.6
West Sepik	114,119	59,168	54,951	51.8
Manus	25,844	13,155	12,689	50.9
New Ireland	65,705	36,349	29,356	55.3
East New Britain	133,530	73,023	60,507	54.7
West New Britain	89,229	48,299	40,930	54.1
North Solomons	128,890	71,578	57,312	55.5
Total	3,006,799	1,573,954	1,421,845	52.3

Note: The total population figures yield a proportion of 109.8 males per 100 females. Compare this with the 1966 census figure of 108.8, the 1971 census figure of 107.7, and the 1973 estimate of 111.7 (Annual Report for Papua New Guinea). The 1981 Australian census found 99.4 males per hundred females.

these obligations were selectively reduced, so that the chief victims of hunger were the very old and the very young, and those least affected were young men in their 20s, followed by young women in the same age group. It is not suggested that Papua New Guineans were often beset by famine; rather it is implicit in Greenough's argument that in any society there is an informal – and perhaps unconscious – ranking of obligations, which becomes explicit and a matter of life and death only in times of extreme stress. In the Papua New Guinea case, female infanticide almost certainly disappeared during the twentieth century, but the underlying son-preference persists. The carrying of sons to clinics is not in itself demographically significant, but it does reveal the values of parents. The outcome of this pervasive preference is stark. It was the fate of women to be over-shadowed by their husbands: it is now their fate also to be over-shadowed by their children.

11
Health education

The public health programme was centralised, technically sophisticated, highly professional, imbued with a sense of urgency, and armed with the most modern drugs. The mood and the approach of its officers precluded the health education of the population at large, since this process would be difficult, might be unnecessary and could yield uncertain benefits. When Robert Black pointed to the increasing salience of health education for the whole society, he pilloried the casual attitudes of the Administration's patrol officers themselves. He showed that they had little interest in hygiene for themselves, and less for the 'boys' who cooked their meals; so they fell victim to avoidable infections.[1] If the Department of Public Health could not change the behaviour of patrol officers, we may assume that village people were even less affected by the diffusion of hygienic ideas. The instructions which did affect villagers were the enforcement of latrine building, and the burial of the dead outside the residential areas of villages and hamlets. On Tubetube island in Milne Bay, the arrival of any government patrol provoked the islanders to the panicky digging of haphazard holes, in the certain knowledge that they would shortly be required to re-inter people or dig pit latrines.[2]

> Theirs not to reason why.
> Theirs but to dig or die.

One category of health workers did have a clear educational brief. Aid post orderlies, the most junior stratum of the health service, were selected for training by fellow villagers. When they returned from training, they depended upon the good will of their peers, so they could hardly invoke criminal sanctions. Furthermore, they could only deliver those services which villagers requested.[3] To be effective, each APO must be thoroughly involved in village affairs; but to retain the confidence of their Australian supervisors, they must seem to remain aloof. In her absorbing account of life in Minj (in the western highlands), Margaret Spencer describes a chance visit to the aid post at nearby Banz:

> Unfortunately, it became clear from various complaints that Aba, the orderly in charge, has become involved locally in such a way that it will be necessary to withdraw him to the hospital at Minj. It would be difficult for any orderly in charge of an aid-post to keep entirely clear of local politics as a position of even minor authority can easily be turned to advantage in many ways. Aba has

a very shrewd and resolute face, with an I-know-where-I'm-going look, and a quietly capable manner.[4]

He needed all his shrewd resolution to satisfy the conflicting demands on his behaviour.

The training of APOs began almost as soon as the war ended, first at Idubada on the outskirts of Port Moresby, and later at several provincial centres. They were expected to spend their lives in the village of their birth, seeking no career beyond that horizon. They would carry out a series of prescribed functions, under supervision from visiting medical assistants and doctors. Accordingly, their training programme was brief, there were no educational pre-requisites, and (at least in principle) even an illiterate could become an APO.[5] They replaced the medical *tultuls*, who lapsed into invisible obscurity, their 1930s training of no further value. By the peak of the programme in the early 1960s, there were about 1,400 APOs at work in the countryside.[6] But their hour was brief: as transport improved, and as better-trained health extension officers became more widely available, APOs were marginalised. By 1970

> In many parts of the country the APO, looked down upon because of his lack of education, inadequate training, and lack of recognition, has lost heart and sees no way to improve his lot. In the last few years, the training standards have been greatly improved, but at the same time the Administration has [temporarily] stopped training orderlies.[7]

Nurse training – for hospital and rural extension work – remained entirely a mission activity until 1953. The tragic explosion of Mount Lamington in the Northern Province of Papua, in 1951, provoked the building of a hospital at Saiho, nearby, where the department trained MCH nurses alongside the general nurses being instructed by the Anglican mission.[8] There the programme lingered in limbo until Port Moresby General Hospital was ready in 1957, and the department could begin more formal education. Mission influence was not sloughed off merely by transferring the programme to Port Moresby. Most of the first students were recruited from mission backgrounds, and so were most of their instructors, including the first Assistant Director for Medical Training (Dr Kenneth Todd) who transferred across from the Kwato mission.[9] The first intake of students included almost equal numbers of men and women, but nursing swiftly became a predominantly female profession, attracting many more women than men into the ranks of the training programme.[10]

One specialism was, from its inception, entirely female: maternal and child health nursing. Sister Betty Crouch, pioneering in this field for the Baptist mission, sought out anyone who was not discouraged by the hardships of that career, with its constant travelling and the absolute requirement of resourcefulness.[11] Dr Joan Refshauge began MCH nurse-training on a more systematic basis during the 1950s. When she drafted her report for 1952–53, she noted with surprise and pleasure a notable enthusiasm amongst native women and girls for the training in welfare work offered ... and trainees readily accept transfer, with the full concurrence of their parents, to places remote from their homes, for purposes of training. The full significance of this development can only be gauged properly in the light of the well known tendency towards conservatism in the native communities.[12]

That 'well known tendency' may be an artifact of anthropology and colonial policy: every opportunity available for nurse training had been seized avidly. As soon as Kwato mission began to seek trainee nurses, during the 1930s, for example, volunteers were forthcoming. Nedulia, for instance,[13] had completed her own family when, in her thirties, she was sufficiently moved by the carnage of unassisted child-birth, and sufficiently impressed by the possibility of averting it, that she trained as a nurse. The rest of her career resembled that of an evangelical *liklik dokta*, constructing her own bush-materials clinic, and if necessary stealing the materials with which to build. Probably the only Papuan New Guinean woman to be decorated during the Pacific War was another Kwato nurse who was not merely brave and resourceful, but *visibly* so.[14] Career women of this kind do not crop up in Papua New Guinea colonial history before the Pacific War, except in Milne Bay during the 1930s – but then Milne Bay was the only district in which the opportunity was presented.[15]

Some problems did crop up in the MCH nurse training scheme. A high proportion of recruits failed to return after their first annual holiday. That tendency persisted, and the training course was re-designed such that a nurse who dropped out after the first of the three years would have acquired many of the practical skills likely to be required in a village community. Dr Refshauge hoped that they would make better wives and mothers as a result.[16] Only a small minority of trainees persevered through a life-time career: most married and had children, and dropped out of the paid work-force at least for a number of years. Nevertheless the medical service did offer the alternative of a career, and created at least the impression of choice for many women who previously had none. Not surprisingly, some women chose a life of salaried and recognised nurturing, rather than unpaid drudgery.[17]

At the beginning of the peace, Gunther deployed a few doctors and nurses, but much larger numbers of European and Papuan medical assistants and *tultuls*. The general trend, made possible by the training programme, was to shift towards four categories of staff: doctors, nurses, health extension officers and APOs. Few of the Papuan medical assistants remained in the department after the war; and the supply of war-time trained European medical assistants gradually dried up. During the 1960s, the training of health extension officers (alongside nurses) steadily became more thorough, providing a supply of intermediate health workers.[18] However, the general improvements in transport and communication, the professionalisation of the department and the mission services, and above all the availability of the refugee European doctors, made for a 'doctor-centred' medical service. Since the refugee doctors had to be considered a stop-gap measure, unlikely to be available in the future, the training of indigenous doctors assumed some urgency.

Gunther's intention at the end of the war was to train Papua New Guineans at every possible level. Given the miserable educational institutions of the previous generation, there was only one appropriate training course available – the Central Medical School at Suva in Fiji, which had been training native medical assistants since the late 1920s, for every dependency in the Anglophone Pacific except New Guinea and Papua. Accordingly, seven young men were despatched to Suva in 1947. The selection might have been more careful: one student was found to have tuberculosis, and another was sent back to a Fijian high school to prepare himself better for the medical course.[19] A third – Albert Maori Kiki – was selected very largely because Bert Speer, that kind-hearted European medical assistant, considered him too bright to remain in domestic service.[20] Some of the students survived and qualified; but the opportunity was closed off when the CMS abruptly raised its entrance standards in 1947, beyond a level which Papua New Guinea's schools could reach. Not until 1952 was it possible to send any more students.[21] Australian medical schools were barred by the same inadequate secondary schooling; and it took several years before the department had the resources and personnel to begin their own medical education at that level.

The Papuan Medical College, which admitted its first candidates to become doctors in 1960, had been teaching nurses and medical assistants for the previous two years in the precincts (actually the animal house and some spare wards) of Port Moresby General Hospital.[22] In these bizarre conditions, the question of making medical education relevant to the needs and circumstances of Papua New Guinea had an obvious point. Much effort was devoted to ensuring social relevance. Sociology in the first year attempted to sketch the context of medical work:

> A person coming from a primitive culture is tremendously curious about the culture of civilisation. By approaching his own culture through the culture of civilisation, primitive society becomes meaningful in a way it could not otherwise have done.[23]

Second year sociology introduced basic sociological concepts; surveyed the evolution of social, political and economic institutions in early modern Europe, Australia, and Papua New Guinea; considered case studies of the reception of health services, and explored the application of sociology to real-life situations. Third year students went on to anthropology:

> As every aspect of primitive life is tied in with attitudes to illness and the curing of disease, an objective study of the former helps the doctor to introduce changes in the latter, and most important of all it helps him to understand and modify the attitudes of his patients based in the magico-religious beliefs of their culture.[24]

In 1966 an element of psychology was added (at third year level). During the fourth year of study, when all students spent three months at the Rural Health Training Centre in Goroka in the eastern highlands, the social science learning was reinforced:

> Family and clan organisation is discussed with the old men, a map is made and a census taken. Each student is given an aspect of the village life to investigate, such as diet, native medicines, the role of magic practitioners, behaviour towards strangers.[25]

Such confidence in the objectivity of the social sciences reads oddly in the 1980s, and in retrospect it could be described as locating Melanesian societies rather arbitrarily in a unilinear and evolutionary framework of human experience. But the programme seems to have worked as a device for describing the social context of therapies. The first three graduates were capped at the end of 1964.

Although the Papuan Medical College was a very small entity, its teaching resources were expanded by calling on consultants (mainly from Australia) to teach segments of the programme, and by involving many members of staff from the Port Moresby General Hospital and from the rest of the Public Health Department. And so matters might have continued if not for the creation of the University of Papua New Guinea. The Currie Commission on Higher Education (of which Dr Gunther was a member) recommended a shortening of the existing programme, leading to a licentiate which the future university would confer. The staff of the college developed a counter-proposal in 1969, whereby the college would become the medical faculty of the university, offering courses towards a full degree. The Minister for Territories rejected their proposal, partly on the grounds that a university faculty would raise standards unnecessarily high, and expenses with them. His rejection provoked 'immediate and widespread reaction from many sections of the community in Papua New Guinea and from distinguished academic and medical figures', and the minister bowed to this pressure.[26] The first appointments were made in 1970, and a full degree course began the following year.

For nearly a generation, therefore, Papua New Guinea has educated most of its own health professionals. An obvious point to make about this achievement is that it eliminated much of the variety of background which characterised health personnel in the 1950s and 1960s. The retirement of the Hungarians and Ukrainians left a void which has been filled by Papua New Guineans, Australians and Britons for the most part. What the later generation of doctors share in common is not national background, but adherence to an agreed set of standards and values. That may seem a bland observation, in view of the issue of educational standards which has persistently racked the medical faculty of the university. To state the issue more crudely than its protagonists do, two general views have been advanced, on the role of medicine in a 'developing country'. One view would be that any divergence from Australian standards and methods is a lowering of those standards, casting a slur on Papua New Guinean capacities. The opposite view would be that Australian standards and procedures can only lead to a cadre of professionals equipped to deal with Australian social and medical circumstances.[27] The resolution of this conflict has usually been to include a very wide range of 'community medicine' subjects in the medical curriculum – but not to threaten the ability of medical graduates to proceed to post-graduate and fellowship studies in Australia or in Britain.[28] The outcome is a thoroughly impressive degree programme, producing a somewhat homogeneous medical graduate.

Homogeneity also perhaps describes the gradual replacement of the old medical assistants (many of whom were de facto general practitioners) and the early APOs, by Health Extension Officers of a more predictable quality. The rapid transformation of transport and communications throughout the country has enabled much variation to be ironed out of health care – and the independence of the medical assistants and APOs to be undermined.

A second consequence may be mentioned in passing. When Black launched his appeal for health education in the late 1950s, he sought a departure from the esoteric style of health administration, and the inclusion of the whole population in the discussion of goals and methods in public health. As we shall see in the following chapters, many doctors took up his cause during the 1960s and 1970s. Yet the outcome in the 1980s is a professional department possessed of a more diffuse body of esoteric information than ever before, and still remote from the general public. Reviewing the work of the Health Extension Officers in 1970, Calvert concluded that

> Hygiene workers do teach many good habits. However ... they must take care to teach only those methods tested locally, or in very similar areas, and shown to actually improve village living conditions. They should honestly assess the results of their teaching and not be content to blame the villagers for any bad effects that follow. There is no doubt that some teaching is actually causing harm to the people it is supposed to help.[29]

What was then (and is now) at issue is not the technical appropriateness of such advice as is given, but its unilinear passage from the professionals who have knowledge, to the populace which allegedly does not. Despite the impressive knowledge possessed by the professionals – or perhaps because of it – well-being is still a condition which is seen to be conferred upon the people, not something which is to be achieved by local initiative.

12
A national health system

By the 1960s, health services were fragmented: each piece the product of historical conditions which were passing away. Each of the major mission societies operated an autonomous health care service, focused on the area where that mission predominated. Within the Public Health Department, the Division of Maternal and Child Health (with its own Deputy Director) ran programmes catering to quite distinct public needs; and the units (waging the campaigns) specialised in the control of one infection each. A District Medical Officer was simultaneously answerable to several regional supervisors of campaign units, and to the hierarchy of the department at large, centred in Port Moresby. If the District Medical Officer was baffled by competing demands on his time and resources, the aid post orderly was even more bewildered by the variety of medical specialists who passed through the village, sometimes offering assistance, sometimes demanding support, and at other times ignoring the aid post entirely.[1]

If the dislocation was most acute in the department, it was in the missions that the strongest arguments were made for integration and a better planned service. One of the architects of integration, Dr Hakan Hellberg, recorded his impressions for the guidance of later historians.[2] He identified several impulses towards change in the late 1960s:

1 Development towards self-government accelerated.
2 National churches started taking over responsibility from overseas mission groups.
3 Increased emphasis was placed on community health.
4 A rapid rise occurred in the cost of medical services.
5 Serious discussion took place about the relevance of medical missionary work or church-based medical activities.
6 Ecumenical contacts between churches increased.

These developments deserve fuller consideration. The pace of constitutional change was mainly determined in Canberra, and was commonly faster than the Papua New Guinean House of Assembly desired. By the mid-1960s, decolonisation was on the political agenda, and missionaries were anxious to transform their structures from foreign-based missions into indigenous and self-governing churches. Some mission workers wondered whether the structure of medical servicing was itself a colonial relic, imposing programmes which the congregations had not requested, and

99

justifying health policy decisions in technical and professional terms without public debate. It was a matter of anticipating the demands of self-governing Papua New Guinea rather than responding to them: it was not until 1972 that the House of Assembly called upon the Administration to 'coordinate and integrate, as far as possible, Government, Mission and other resources for Health Services in the Territory'.[3]

Implicit in the shift from mission to church organisation, was the fear of saddling new churches with financial and administrative responsibilities beyond their capacity, and the expectation that a self-governing nation would seek closer control over social services. During the late 1960s and 1970s therefore, the missions and churches surrendered control over their school systems.[4] It would have been anomalous to retain health services, when even the centre-pieces of the mission communities were being made over. In any event, the churches assumed (correctly, as it turned out) that church members would be well represented in the emerging indigenous administration.

The increasing emphasis upon community medicine, which will be considered in the next chapter, added to the pressure for institutional change. At least as important was the impact of increasing costs. This world-wide problem affected the missions acutely, since the department (with its ever-increasing budget) could offer specialist services and training far beyond the reach of the missions. The latter were becoming, de facto, subordinate to the department through sheer technical capacity. The autonomy of each mission, already undermined by reliance on departmental subsidies for work performed to departmental specifications, seemed increasingly hollow.

By long tradition, mission health workers helped to stretch the mission budgets by accepting salaries lower than their departmental counterparts – and below the level of the subsidy paid to the missions for their labour. This was meet, right, and the bounden duty of *missionaries*, but unfairly burdensome for indigenous workers. Reviewing the sources of his unease, the mission doctor Peter Strang pointed to the anomaly:

> Church Aid Post Orderlies were working for $150.00 per year and having to send their children to High School on this wage (with fees at $60.00 per year for one child). Government or Local Government Council-employed Order-lies were receiving $500.00 per year. Qualified nurses and Sisters in Church employment were receiving $150.00 per year, when in Government service they were receiving over $1,000.00 [In the case of his United Church hospital] this meant that we were running Iruna on about $5,000.00 per year ... One thing it did help us to do and that was to get involved with the Local Government Council and the community and have them contribute. This experience helped us all immensely. We also turned our Church Aid Posts over to the Local Government Council.[5]

Through departmental subsidies, self-sacrifice, and reliance on community support, the mission services could survive but this ad hoc arrangement cast doubt on the distinctiveness of medical missionary work, as it became a means of subsidising services planned, approved and supervised by the state. And all the time the old fiefdoms of the missions were crumbling.[6] The issue of high school fees, for example, became salient because the near-monopoly once enjoyed by the missions was yielding to a fast-expanding government Department of Education. Rapidly improving transport brought mission and departmental staff into closer interaction – and pointed up the disparities in their incomes. The same transport revolution undermined the old justification for a self-sufficient mission health service, providing every health need for an isolated community. And the same revolution permitted the churches – in an era of ecumenical tolerance – to meet and to recognise their shared problems.

The first meeting of medical missions was held in 1965. They then met annually, and formed the Churches Medical Council (CMC). The agenda always addressed training programmes – not for doctors, since the department alone could afford such a programme, but for community health workers, who were seen to be the churches' distinctive contribution to the nation's health. The departmental grant-in-aid scheme was always on the agenda as well. And increasingly there were particular issues of rationalisation in the context of liaison with the department.[7] As these questions became more common, and an ad hoc resolution seemed unwise, the CMC appointed Dr Hellberg (from the World Council of Churches) as a consultant in negotiations with the department.[8] By that time – 1972, the eve of self-government – the House of Assembly had added its voice to the demand for rationalisation and integration.

Negotiations with the department proceeded smoothly. There were personal and professional connections between the department and the CMC, since several officers of the department had first worked in the missions, and all authorities could see the sense of better coordination. During the previous twenty years, standards of treatment and preferred techniques had largely been standardised in any case.[9] Technical changes helped to underline the need for organisational change. The trend towards domiciliary care for TB and leprosy patients, for instance, made the specialist isolation hospitals redundant, and it made obvious sense to transform them into district health centres. More fraught were the decisions to resolve the duplication of hospital facilities, usually (but not always) confirming the departmental hospital and requiring the mission hospital to reduce its range of services.[10] A common method of resolving such issues, was a departmental contract to an existing mission organisation, to provide an agreed range of services within a given region, from an established hospital or health centre.[11] That device retained something of the ethos of the mission service, and its commitment to a community – while relieving it of staggering financial burdens and enabling its health workers to receive the 'going rate' for their skills.

Underpinning these negotiations was a vaguely egalitarian sense, often expressed in the belief that the twilight of colonialism was also the dawn of a more democratic and rational era. Nearly a century of ad hoc development of fragmented health services had created a pattern of over-servicing of some areas and under-servicing of others, glued together by the centralism of decision-making in Canberra. The over-riding concern of the new administration which took shape in Port Moresby was to find some new way of holding together a highly disparate series of communities. To summarise a complex political story, the national government resolved upon the construction of strong provincial governments, largely in order to head off Bougainville's threatened secession; and the precedent of provincial government was then extended to every one of the nineteen districts of the old colonial administration.[12]

The consequences for the administration of public health were paradoxical. By about 1973, integration of medical services had been substantially achieved, and the earlier decisions consolidated into the National Health Plan of that year.[13] No sooner was this achieved, than pressure mounted for re-fragmentation, or provincialism. Those pressures were not met by the new pattern of hospitals, whereby every province had precisely one provincial general hospital, and many sub-provinces a health centre. Despite extreme reluctance within the newly localised Health Department headquarters to delegate functions to local authorities, it was impossible for the department to stand out against provincialism. In 1984, a bureaucratic putsch replaced the centralists and cleared the way for the decentralisation of several functions to provincial health authorities.[14]

The mood of the late-colonial years also favoured self-reliance, a diffuse ambition which encompassed autonomy for the provinces, but also aspired to reduce the links of dependence upon a variety of Australian institutions and a very large annual subvention from Canberra towards the national budget.[15] The Papuan Medical College, which became the medical faculty of the new university, and the nursing and health extension officer training institutions, enabled Papua New Guinea to train its own health personnel (albeit at the cost of inflating the annual budget support) apart from the continuing need to send students abroad for post-graduate and specialist education. To help with planning, the Health Department commissioned the stocktaking of resources and statement of problems, which was published as *The diseases and health services of Papua New Guinea*.[16] The rationalisation of services and strict budgeting could stretch those resources to some extent: yet there was certain to be continuing reliance on Australian research services. The first casualty of tight budgeting would have been medical research. This outcome was avoided very largely by the channelling of Australian and other medical scientists through the Institute of Medical Research in Goroka and Madang, which imaginatively harnessed the enthusiasm and skill of foreign research workers to health problems identified by local authorities.

Reliance upon overseas-based researchers is a risky strategy, although the risk may be calculated and may be justified. In 1945, when *kuru* was identified in a remote region of the highlands, Director Gunther intended to delegate the research into this devastating disease to his colleagues at the Walter and Eliza Hall Institute of Medical Research in Melbourne. He was peremptorily pre-empted by Dr Carleton Gajdusek, who invoked the argument that as New Guinea was a United Nations Trust Territory, it was improper to restrict research access to an Australian institution.[17] Gajdusek was vindicated (and won a Nobel Prize) when he was able to show that *kuru* was a long-incubating virus, the first to be demonstrated in humans. Retrospectively, Gunther acknowledged that only Gajdusek, with the North American research resources at his disposal, could have accomplished this feat.

That episode may have helped to create the climate in which Papua New Guinea later became the preferred field-trial region for research into malaria vaccines. By the late 1980s, three international consortia were involved in the pursuit of a successful vaccine, to counteract the remarkable recovery of malaria on a world scale since the 1960s.[18] Whether Papua New Guinea's medical authorities are able to control these three consortia, with their impressive commercial backing, research resources and international ambitions, remains to be seen. If the risk has been well calculated, Papua New Guineans may become the first people in history to enjoy a vaccine for an endemic disease; so the risks of field trials may prove to be justified, and the 'open-door' strategy vindicated again.

The creation of a self-reliant and integrated national health service has not been a neat operation. The autonomy of mission services has disappeared, leaving behind enclaves of health workers still united by a common ethos; but it has been replaced by a national health care system which has delegated a very wide array of functions to 19 provincial governments of uneven administrative quality. Links between the Papua New Guinea health care system and Australian institutions largely persist, though much less formally than before: Australia remains the most common location for post-graduate education, Australian research workers are closely involved in (for example) the development of the malaria vaccine, and Australian standards of teaching and nursing and treatment are often implicitly assumed to be appropriate in Papua New Guinea. Perhaps the most important sense in which a national health care system has evolved, is the integration of the Health Department into the new national bureaucracy, as one of the great spending departments which compete for annual funds instead of submitting project proposals to Canberra to be judged in isolation from the rest of the national economy.

But if the institutional transformation of the Health Department has been incomplete and in some respects messy, it has accomplished some goals which are perhaps not sufficiently remarked. Much of the dedication of the old mission services persists, without being disruptive. The department continues to attract skilled overseas workers, at least for some years of high endeavour before they settle to conventional careers in their home countries.[19] Doctors and nurses of impressive calibre are trained within the country, yet without loss of international credentials.[20] An active research programme continues, despite the lack of funds to make it absolutely a national research effort. Although financial accountability is pitifully weak, and in some provinces this undermines the health extension programmes,[21] for the most part the services are still made available at an impressive standard. The transition from inchoate colonialism to a more orderly independence was a potential health hazard, and the risky transition has been managed.

13
Primary health care

The ideas and techniques of medical care between the wars could be grouped together under the rubric of 'tropical medicine', an organising principle which gave those ideas a general coherence. The massive expansion of medical knowledge and drugs during the 1940s burst the limits of that organising principle: so many infections could be prevented or cured, that medical administrators need no longer rely on quarantine and segregation to defend the health of small enclaves of well-being. Scragg describes the post-war years as the 'curative era'.[1] The great campaigns of those years, when western medicine took the offensive against specific infections, asserted that tropical people need no longer suffer more intensely than temperate societies.

The emergence of a new organising principle lagged behind the technical changes which made it necessary. Meanwhile, medical planners were abandoning their earlier models of health and disease. They were responding not only to a more sophisticated epidemiology, which observed that much 'tropical' ill-health was a consequence of poverty rather than physical environment.[2] They also responded to the political independence of many tropical colonies. The social tendency of tropical medicine – to protect privileged minorities and to acquiesce in the morbidity of the majority – jarred against the rhetoric of newly independent governments.[3] There was also the intriguing example of China's barefoot doctors, and the collaboration of traditional Chinese and modern western specialists. The outcome of new perceptions and opportunities was the strategy of primary health care.

Like tropical medicine before it, primary health care is a strategic vision which commands allegiance but defies implementation. Gee's useful precis describes four elements of the primary health care approach:

essential health care made accessible to everyone in the country;
care given in a way acceptable to individuals, families and the community and requiring their full participation;
care provided at a cost the community and the country can afford;
that primary health care forms an integral part of the country's health system and of the overall social and economic development of the country.[4]

The measures justified by this ideology are legion: indigenous control over policy and programmes, nationally or parochially; a sharp re-direction of resources from curative to preventive effort; and the subordination of therapists to the demands of consumers. Primary health care is not so much a programme as a virtuous state of mind, meaning quite different things to its various supporters.

Some of the new ideas were set out by Dr Maurice King of Makerere in Uganda, in response to much the same dilemma which confronted his counterparts in Papua New Guinea. So long as his work was confined to the general hospital, he could do substantially what he would have done in any metropolitan hospital. As a doctor in the field, however, he found that there were no guidelines on how to make the best use of very limited resources. His *Medical care in developing countries*[5] focused his colleagues' attention on the issues which called for resolution; and his more combative 'Medicine in red and blue'[6] addressed the political dimension of adapting western medicine to a quite different social and health milieu. These ideas were flagged in the editorial columns of the *Papua New Guinea Medical Journal*[7] even before the final text of *Medical care* was published. Together with Bryant's *Health and the developing world*,[8] this new work stressed the social context more than the technical content of medical work; and they were fed into the community medicine curriculum of the Papuan Medical College and its successor, the medical faculty of the university.[9]

Some medical planners were avid for these new ideas. In 1966, Robert Black addressed a medical audience in Port Moresby, and posed the question 'Has it all been worthwhile? – measurement of the results of effort in medicine'. The editor of the *Medical Journal* at least considered this as a revolutionary call to arms. Admitting the possibility that 'sixty years of conscientious activity have been a long and costly mistake, leading to an ingrained emphasis on therapeutics', he suggested that a more productive approach would be 'to ask local government authorities to share the burden of decision as to how money shall be spent on health in their areas, and to underwrite more of the expense'.[10] That response was shared (as we have seen) by many of the more thoughtful mission doctors of the 1960s, who visualised parochial communities helping to draft policies, plan programmes, fund them, and implement them as well.[11]

Other writers on medical policy and practice found rather different ideas to please them in the rich variety suddenly made available. Medical administrators (less inclined than teachers to relish apocalyptic ideas) found it useful in their search for improved forms of organisation, and a better balance between 'specialists and spraymen' within the departmental budget.[12] So widely did these new prescriptions infuse and inform the medical profession, that primary health care was enshrined in the 1974–78 National Health Plan.

But this body of ideas was easier to enshrine than to implement. The period of the first National Health Plan coincided with the collapse of local government councils across the country, as provincial governments were established.[13] Provincial bureaucracies were not the kind of face-to-face parochial meetings which the mission doctors had pre-supposed. That was a difficulty in itself, and it sharpened a further difficulty. The necessary focus of a community-based health care system is the village-based health-worker – in this instance the aid post orderly. The APO is the only possible channel of technical information, interpreter of local enthusiasms, and translator of dreams into health-giving reality. The APO is the essential link between technology and society. One of the widespread phenomena of the 1970s was a break-down in relations between the political centre and the rural localities. The APOs became isolated from the sources of technical information, the planners of health projects, and the resources to work with.[14] Of all the possible dimensions of a primary health care system, the full participation of rural communites was ruled out.

A great many useful and health-giving measures do not, of course, require popular participation. An impressive and unusual project of this era was the banning of feeding bottles. It was unusual because many third world governments have not been able to resist the blandishments of baby-food pushers, and it was possible because technical advice to politicians did not have to be compromised by public debate among the users of feeding bottles. It is quite likely that this prohibition has averted a great deal of child sickness.[15] By contrast, MCH workers on their rural patrols have been profoundly affected by the demand for statistical reporting and the meeting of numerical targets. Probably this has led to an efficient delivery of a stated quota of injections, but the patrols have become ritualised to the point where nutritional advice and ante-natal care have withered.[16] Since the great majority of maternity risk factors can be anticipated by timely interviews, even without physical inspection, this ritualisation has allowed a high maternal mortality rate to persist.[17] Even more inefficient is the process of planning and installing wells for clean water (in itself a wholly admirable idea), with so little discussion among consumers that most wells quickly fall into disrepair.[18] Much of the 1970s health work therefore is open to precisely the same objections as the old centrally-directed campaigns against specific infections: there are limits to the effectiveness of those measures which really require local support.

Many hopes were pinned upon the education of doctors and nurses, to carry the banner of primary health care into the professions. A certain level of resistance was predictable, and predicted:

> But if we [were to] spend so much of the limited time available in a Medical Course on practical problems in administration, sociology, health education, public health, shall we not be accused of producing second-rate, non-scientific doctors?[19]

Yes, they would be so accused. Bravely, the faculty held out for an education relevant to the circumstances of most doctors in Papua New Guinea, despite the suspicion of some students that a different education must be an inferior one. Yet the full vision of the primary health care advocates was not entirely absorbed into the medical curriculum for doctors. Equally important, with independence and urbanisation came the opportunity for some medical graduates to branch out into private practice. That slippage has been less than might have been expected,[20] yet every private practitioner in urban or mining enclaves diminishes the possibility of equal access within a community-based health care system. In brief, the strategy and its moral imperatives cut across the grain of the day-to-day reality of therapists and their patients.

To re-direct health services when the village-based workers were isolated, when doctors were sceptical, and when Health Extension Officers and doctors were mutually suspicious,[21] required medical administration of an exceptional quality. In practice, at the time of self-government a new cadre of medical administrators was plunged into authority, and immediately forced to grapple with the question of decentralisation of functions to the new provincial governments. The new administrators, often graduates of Fiji or the Papuan Medical College, and possibly over-awed by their university-trained staff, naturally clung to procedures and hierarchies which had evidently worked in the past. A later enquiry describes the loss of control and purpose:

> Health services comprise basically hospitals, community services (mainly rural) and special programmes. Rural services were decentralised [to provincial governments] in 1978 but further decentralisation was resisted by the Department of Health, which insisted on dual control of remaining functions. This meant a continuation of vertical chains of command down to the provincial level. Before independence this vertical structure was effective, being based on strong management and planning, with direct control of events in the provinces. With dual control (of much expanded health services) however, the structure impeded effective functioning of hospitals and special programmes. The national department itself lost control of events. This resulted in an almost complete breakdown of information systems and analysis, an absence of sensible planning or clear policy guidelines for the national and provincial departments to follow, and an inability to comply with the national planning process regarding finance and manpower.[22]

If we refer back to Kingsley Gee's description of primary health care, it becomes clear that it had not been implemented during the 1970s. Improved transport and the aid post building programme had certainly brought more and more people within walking distance of some health care[23] – but of uncertain and uneven quality. Care was given in a way acceptable to health workers and statistics-gatherers, but not necessarily to consumers, who did not participate in planning or implementing (or funding) these activities. Given the extreme dependence of the state upon foreign aid, it is doubtful whether the community or the country was affording such care as it received. And health care was manifestly unrelated to the overall social and economic development of the country. The achievements were often impressive, but they were not a primary health care programme.[24]

Life expectancy – the simplest measure of health – has increased markedly through the 1970s.[25] Health plans also demand equality of well-being; so it is appropriate to review progress towards that equality. In particular, we may enquire about equality across environmental regimes, across social circumstances, across generations, and between the sexes.

The national census of 1980, the most thorough yet attempted, is the basis for estimates of life expectancy on a provincial basis, from 1971 to 1980. The estimates suggest almost universal improvement. Men and women in all provinces can expect to live longer than ever before. The wide difference between the most morbid and the most healthy province in 1971 had shrunk appreciably by 1980.[26] Even allowing for error in estimating ages, the figures suggest a gratifying 'equalisation upwards' in living standards. But the provincial basis of data collection conceals a significant element of inequality. Every province includes a range of environments: no province covers *only* the highlands fringe region, which is a zone of special hazard and hardship. Detailed studies of particular communities in this zone[27] describe a double disadvantage. On one hand, roads do not serve these areas nearly as well as they serve areas of cash crop or mineral production, so that extension services are thin. On the other hand, old hazards persist, in the form of malaria, dysentery, and malnutrition, reducing human resistance to every other infection.

Two studies illustrate the range of health conditions across environments. Scragg's account of Lemankoa village on Buka Island in the North Solomons describes the most favourable impact of the gamut of health services.[28] An 'epidemic era' persisted until 1942, in which high fertility was matched by high mortality, and the population fluctuated around a stable base line. The impact of war was especially severe, so that population declined until 1947; but that disaster was followed swiftly by a

> curative era with an increasing population due to a rapid fall in mortality caused by the paternalistic application of modern lifesaving medicines by village health workers through a village aid post but with increased fertility due to the destruction of traditional family planning practices and attitudes.

The fourth era of health care – preventive – dawned in 1960:

> with a more rapidly increasing population, and a further decline in mortality due to the application on a district and national scale of disease prevention programmes but with stable fertility until the 1970s when socio-economic development has started a fertility decline.

Always accessible to the most up-to-date medical programmes, to cash crop opportunities, and to education through the missions, Lemankoa is untypical of Papua New Guinea. However, its experience

> indicate[s] the potential for mortality reduction and for national fertility transition [to low fertility and low mortality] if effective curative and preventive services are matched with economic and social development in the rural village.

Summarised into life expectancy rates, Lemankoa people born between 1927 and 1942 could expect to live to 22 (for men) and 25 (for women): their grandchildren born after 1960 could expect to live to 64 or 68.

By contrast, people living in the North Fly region, close to the Indonesian border, were brought to the country's attention only when the Ok Tedi gold and copper mine was planned in the late 1970s. The first survey, by a World Health Organisation team, was puzzled:

> The severity of clinical disease appears to be less than expected, and to vary from area to area. Malaria is everywhere the principal cause of ill-health. Filariasis shows a patchy and unexpected distribution and severity . . . Neither leprosy nor tuberculosis is a major problem . . . Malnutrition is clinically obvious in only a few places, and is not associated with food shortages, though anaemia which is quite common is probably due principally to deficient iron intake. Skin diseases are a major cause of morbidity. Lower respiratory tract disease is common and debilitating . . . hookworm . . . are perhaps less prevalent than in similar ecosystems . . . The cause of the increased death rate in middle age has not been identified, but is expected to be related to virus diseases especially influenza.[29]

A detailed study of a small community confirms the short life-span, high fertility matched by high mortality, and little visible ill-health precisely because the sick do not survive to be counted.[30] By comparison with Lemankoa, the North Fly population – on the eve of a massive mining development in their midst – were still languishing in the 'epidemic era' awaiting the arrival of organised health care. Professor Lourie's research team documented the short life expectancy of the Wopkaimin society, and

> has abundantly confirmed much of this ill-health, recording in particular hyperendemicity of malaria . . . widespread anaemia, and a crude infant mortality rate of 230 per thousand live births. A group such as the Wopkaimin has been living . . . in a supremely delicate ecological balance with the natural environment. The inevitable cost has been a high disease load and infant mortality, and low life expectancy.

To the unequal conditions of environment, colonialism added the unequal social conditions of urbanisation and rural resettlement. Julian Tudor Hart's 'inverse care law' was formulated to describe the distribution of health care in Britain, but it has a wider application. It points to a persistent tendency for the best care to go to those who least need it:

> The force that creates and maintains the inverse care law is the operation of the market, and its cultural and ideological superstructure which has permeated the thought and directed the ambitions of our profession during all its modern history. The more health services are removed from the force of the market, the more successful we can be in redistributing care away from its 'natural' distribution in a market economy . . .[31]

The 'inverse care law' can be tested against the very different conditions of contemporary Papua New Guinea,[32] because the free market is not yet developed. The market is constrained by provincial governments, which ensure some re-distribution away from the urban centre of Port Moresby, and it is curtailed by the missionary enthusiasm of a proportion of the doctors and nurses in the country, so that the inverse care law does not enjoy a free hand. Despite these constraints, urban consumers are better served than their rural cousins. The expansion of private medical practice from the 1970s worked entirely to the advantage of urban people. And even within the government service, it has been impossible to prevent Port Moresby General Hospital from accumulating a disproportionate share of resources and staff.[33] Since the hospital is usually the first resort of urban patients (whereas rural patients more commonly consult an aid post orderly first, or a health sub-centre) urban people enjoy more direct access to the best available services. As in every other social service, the rural areas have the highest priority – urban areas merely have the best resources.

Urbanisation remains a small phenomenon in Papua New Guinea. A more diffuse re-orientation of people's lives can be found in the commercialisation of rural production. Plantations were the commonest expression of this trend until the 1960s. Since then, more people's lives have been re-shaped by rural resettlement schemes, usually centred upon nucleus estates committed to cultivating and processing a single tropical tree crop for export.[34] People brought from over-crowded regions to these settlements have been employed either as wage labourers on the nucleus estate itself, or as holders of blocks of land dedicated to the supervised production of the crop. Already nutritionists and health extension workers have observed disturbing indications of under-nutrition among the settler families; and the large families who grow to adulthood on blocks designed to sustain a nuclear family, will presumably suffer a declining standard of living in the future. Even in the supervised resettlement schemes, it has proved difficult to organise the local health committees which could alleviate some of the avoidable health problems.[35]

Despite the reassurance of the provincial demographic evidence, therefore, it seems clear that the old (environmental) sources of unequal health persist, and that new (social) forms create new inequities in health care. Well-being may be increasing, but it is increasing unequally from region to region, and from social class to class.

An enduring enthusiasm of health workers has been the reduction of the infant mortality rate (a feature emphasised in both the Lemankoa and the North Fly study, and in virtually every other survey). A paradoxical consequence of successful campaigns against infant mortality is that the Papua New Guinea population is constantly becoming younger, even though life expectancy has stretched. Whether this is a consequence of MCH patrols injecting and vaccinating children, or of the diffusion of better nutrition and living standards, is too large a question to address here.[36] It is sufficient to observe that the younger the citizen, the greater the benefit from health programmes.

Although the whole population lives longer, it remains true that men outnumber women by a wide margin. Happy and healthy Lemankoa, enjoying some of the best social and therapeutic conditions in the country, has relatively equal numbers of men and women.[37] The only whole province which has more female than male inhabitants is the Southern Highlands, which is also the largest reservoir of migration. Here the predominance of women is the measure of the province's under-development, just as the predominance of men in Port Moresby indicates relative over-development. The implication of this population distribution is serious for health projections, because the concentration of health services in urban areas and in regions of cash crop production brings men rather than women within the umbrella of the best health facilities. Women rather than men remain exposed to the most hazardous environments. To take one element of the health care system as an example, we have noted that medical assistance in child birth is rarely available in rural areas. In those urban (and some rural) areas where there is fairly easy access to birth centres and hospitals, they are well patronised. Maternal mortality rates in urban areas are about 2 per thousand deliveries: in remote rural areas they are thought to be about 20 per thousand.[38] It is at least possible that rural women would resort to birth centres if they were equally accessible.[39] Maternal mortality is not, however, the only discriminator between male and female well-being. Robin Hide's study of ageing in one rural part of the highlands argues that women age more swiftly than men, within the same society and environment;[40] and there is no reason to consider his sample untypical.[41] When Michael Young discovered that parents were twice as likely to take their sons to a clinic than their daughters (see chapter 4), he asked some of his Goodenough Island informants for their explanation.

> Our grandfathers used to call women 'bouncing coconuts'. They do not stay with their fathers but leave to go to some other group. But men are different. They do not leave the place where they were born . . . Men are the owners of the village, its inheritors. They are like houseposts but women are like bouncing coconuts. Men marry and look after their own villages; women marry and look after other men's villages . . . Today we put it this way. If a girl is sick her father will say it is of no importance. But if his son is sick he will say to his wife 'Go and take him for medicine'. He will take it and get better, and his father will say 'Good, for he is my heir'.[42]

So long as that priority persists, nutrition and medical care and education will reflect and reinforce gender inequality.

In the confused groping towards a primary health care strategy, the medical authorities had many circumstances in their favour. Governments of the 1970s were committed, at least rhetorically, to redistribution and participation: they now favour increased production first, and redistribution later.[43] The medical profession was (and largely remains) highly motivated towards general welfare and equal access: they were (and largely remain) insulated from the direct play of a free market in health care. Papua New

Guinea had one of the most powerful traditions of parochial participation. The opportunity has not evaporated, but diminished.

During the 1970s also, it became distressingly clear that – whatever the personal motivation of health workers – the structure of contemporary medicine itself was an obstacle to popular participation in health programmes. Maddocks concluded his impressive analysis of medicine and colonialism with the observation that medical technology can never be fully mastered in a developing country, because it evolves and develops as fast as the old skills can be transferred.

> And Medicine is even more persuasive and subtle than other technologies in its colonial role because even within the colonial power itself, Medicine has a colonial structure – its institution and its services being, on the whole, designed and administered by doctors to their specifications and to meet their own peculiar needs.[44]

A benign and paternalist Health Department could still enable the whole of Papua New Guinea's people to reach the levels of well-being enjoyed by Lemankoa. But this ambition is more likely to be achieved through paternalist administration, than by primary health care. As in Aboriginal Australia,[45] so in Papua New Guinea: the social distance between therapists and patients is a persistent obstacle to popular participation in the health programmes.

If we ask why a primary health care strategy has not been implemented, the fault probably does not lie with individual doctors or medical planners, nor with politicians and the political structure, but in the concept itself. Primary health care shares some attributes with the organising principle which it replaced – tropical medicine. In each case the strategic vision is a series of moral exhortations rather than a programme of action. It is a state of mind, not an agenda. And in a sense it does not much matter that primary health care is an impossible dream, so long as practitioners believe in it. In the name of primary health care, many doctors and nurses have performed heroic and altruistic prodigies. This is because the strategy conforms with George Bernard Shaw's description of any prescriptive ideology: it is a strategy to which people will dedicate their lives, because they cannot fully grasp it. And they cannot grasp it because it is not itself coherent.

14
The past and the future

Past performance is our only guide in suggesting how people might extract the greatest benefit from the resources at their disposal. The historical records of medical services are irritatingly incomplete: they tantalise but do not satisfy. The distinction between 'well-being' and 'ill-being' is itself arbitrary. Then medical officers record the information which happens to interest them, and historians compound the problem by selecting such information as seems significant in the light of present conditions and concerns. That arbitrary, narrow and doctor-centred record is nevertheless our only evidence on which to pass judgement and to guide policy.

Medical historians explain the evolution of policies and programmes by seeking change within the medical profession, or by reference to change in the wider society and economy. Writers about Papua New Guinea have located the initiative in one of four ways. The locomotive of change may be Great Doctors, or the medical profession on a world scale; or medical services may spring from the political economy of the country, or from the interests of the colonial authorities who (in the case of Papua New Guinea) paid most of the medical bills.

Great Doctor theories of public health excite not only doctors, who enjoy some vicarious glory, but also scholars who prefer simple explanations. At least five doctors have seemed to command events in Papua New Guinea almost in Wagnerian fashion. MacGregor understood and described health hazards in the 1890s so lucidly that he could almost have been the initiator of the primary health care ideas of the present generations. Sixty years before the world was ready for his prescriptions, however, his actual impact upon health in British New Guinea was minimal, and his strategic vision was not adopted by the profession. His contemporary, Robert Koch, who brought the good news of quinine from Europe to German New Guinea, helped to rescue that morbid outpost of imperialism: but that information would surely have reached Rabaul by some other route. Walter Strong, presiding over Papua's health for a generation, certainly squeezed a remarkable amount of service out of a shrinking budget. He was not the prime mover, however. He shared Governor Murray's enthusiasms – and blind spots – and he owed to Murray the patronage in Canberra and Sydney, which made his work possible.

In a less appealing fashion, Cilento presents himself as a man of destiny, the generalissimo of the New Guinea service, the instrument of

Australian endeavour in tropical medicine, and a star performer on the Australian and international stages. His influence may well have been decisive, for instance in preventing New Guineans from studying medicine. Australian commitment to tropical medicine, however, was short-lived. Cilento was in any event imbued with the military values and virtues (and vices) of his generation. In his absence, it is doubtful whether medical strategy would have been very different, and unlikely that New Guineans would have been appreciably sicker (or healthier) than they were in reality.

John Gunther has the strongest claim of any, to be a prime mover. He was such fun to interview, and his abrasive manner so woefully failed to conceal his compassion, that this rough Australian diamond captured the imagination of health analysts. He did mobilise, equip, and inspire an ebullient department. A lesser man – like some of his contemporary heads of departments – could certainly have fumbled his opportunities. The mood and resources (and strategic confusion) of the Commonwealth Government presented an opportunity, but the effective department was not merely the consequence of Canberra's willingness to fund it. Gunther was charismatic.

The substantial objection to Great Doctor theories is not personal: it is the theory's assumption that doctors are central to public health processes. The lesson to be learned from Europe in the nineteenth century, and from every society in the twentieth, is that doctors are less important to well-being than sanitary engineers, public works foremen, and nurses. We can usefully recall Robert Black's perception that doctors neither create health nor eradicate disease, but cure individual sufferers. Even in their role as policy-makers, doctors are constrained by public finance, by policies laid down outside the Public Health Departments, by public attitudes, and by the state of medical technology. If doctors dominate the sphere of individual illness, they only appear to command the stage of public health.

The state of medical technology has been determined internationally. It is hardly an exaggeration to suggest that a practitioner in Peru in 1900 prescribed the same remedies as a practitioner in Papua at the same time, and that their grandchildren in 1980 were again of one mind. Within a monolithic profession, there have been a few local peculiarities. There was an interval of a few years between the demonstration that beri-beri was the consequence of vitamin deficiency, and its application in New Guinea and in Papua early this century. By the 1940s, even that interval had been eliminated. The evolution of ideas and therapeutic regimes within the profession has had profound and swift consequences in the periphery. Thus the isolation of tropical medicine as a distinct set of ideas and techniques in the 1890s, affected the training and outlook of doctors in Melanesia by about the turn of the century. International conferences for the Pacific islands during the 1920s, and the correlation of quarantine information, reinforced the internationalism of medical practice between the wars. And the coordination of a global medical strategy by the World Health Organisation since the 1940s has set the seal on international professionalism.

Local medical planners often found this irksome. MacGregor was uneasy about the way in which tropical medicine evolved. Murray and Strong resented Cilento's prominence at international gatherings in the 1920s. Gunther refused to be constrained by current orthodoxy in treating tuberculosis, still less by the inhibition against recruiting Australian specialists, and least of all by the South Pacific Commission's pretension to coordinate all South Pacific health services. Yet it was difficult to insist upon Papua New Guinean autonomy in health matters: any resistance to international medical opinion had to be strenuous and cunning, and few issues were worth the trouble.

In spite of sustained pressure to conform to professional standards and procedures, Papua New Guinea medical services were never *simply* the local expression of international strategies. For one thing, administrators did not have the resources to implement international ideas immediately, or absolutely, on every occasion. In the first years of this century, medical services could reach no further than the little expatriate enclaves. Between the wars, Papuan poverty reduced the medical establishment to a skeleton. Briefly during the 1920s Australian medical politics invigorated the New Guinea health services, but interest waned and resources were stretched during the 1930s to cover the newly-explored highlands region. Postwar prosperity in Australia, combined with the strengthening of the federal government, financed the new campaigns of the 1950s. Medical strategies coincided with the health of the colonial state and the volume of finance at its disposal. The local milieu had at least some influence on the quantity, the quality, and the general direction of medical services.

Colonialism was the matrix in which modern medical services emerged in Papua New Guinea, and there is some value in relating those services to the interests which dominated the colonial state. Maddocks shows very elegantly that many medical institutions bear comparison with the structures of colonial authority. Doctors and hospitals resemble district commissioners and district headquarters, each imposing hegemony over the surrounding population. A political economy approach would push the analogy further, and read the programmes of the medical services as expressions of the economic interests of dominant groups within the colonial economy. That perception has some explanatory power, since medical policy often reflected colonial strategy. While the colonial economies were dominated by gold prospectors and planters (and their labour lines), the main thrust of the small medical services was to strengthen the managers and their workers, while the bulk of the population was kept at arm's length. The need of the colonial economy for an expanded and more productive population in the 1950s, is clearly related to the great public health campaigns of that era. Towards the end of the colonial era, some doctors sought to transform the relationships between health workers and the people, and they thought that these reforms were analogous to 'decolonisation'. With self-government, the medical services were brought under the influence of the planning arm of the new state; and Public Health shared the discomfort of all the big spending departments in their new subordination to the national government.

In these very general terms, the linkage between the colonial state and health services is clear enough. To push the argument further, however, does not add more light. Papua New Guinea did not have an orthodox colonial economy during most of the colonial era. The colonial state was not so much an expression of capitalist interests, as an extension of the Australian state over a region of strategic sensitivity. Papua New Guinea had little commercial value to Australia, and attracted little private capital until the 1960s and beyond. More often than not, medical services relied on external funding: that was always true in mission medical services, and it was clearly the case during the heroic 1950s and 1960s.

The historical record also yields uncomfortable evidence against the political economy approach. If anyone personified merchant and agricultural capital in New Guinea, it was Walter Lucas. The former manager of the trading company Burns, Philp & Co., and a member of Billy Hughes' kitchen cabinet in the 1920s, he also headed the Expropriation Board in New Guinea. We have observed his clear statement of the interests of capital in a medical service of a particular kind; we have counted the money which he transferred to medical purposes; and we have seen Colonel Honman sweep away the funds and ignore the policy prescription. Honman was an indifferent doctor, an erratic administrator, and politically marginal. If so feeble a force as Honman could resist so powerful an influence as Lucas, then the political economy approach is fatally flawed.

The breezy Rockefeller agent Sam Lambert is worth observing in this context. He won the support of planters for his hookworm campaign, not because he delivered a vigorous labour line, but because he promised to do so. In his reading of the relationship between medicine and politics, the game was to win political support for a programme which was developed purely as a medical enterprise. A generation later John Gunther read medical politics in much the same light. Gunther also wooed the planters for his great campaigns, by appealing to their self-interest – and with scant regard for literal accuracy. He treated the federal Australian government in much the same fashion – it was a constituency to be won by phrasing policy proposals so as to touch particular sensibilities. Gunther allowed Canberra and the planters the illusion of initiating policy – provided that they encouraged him to do what he had in mind in the first place. Professional analysis came first; then followed policy discussions which the doctors must win if they watched their language; then came the implementation of programmes (by medical professionals). Given the towering prestige of the medical profession, and the unwillingness of planters or public servants to overturn professional judgments, the medical authorities enjoyed a real measure of autonomy in proposing, developing and implementing health programmes.

What, then, were the real determinants of public policy? We are entitled to look to Australia for part of the answer. First, the Papua New Guinea *Government* had a salience in determining health policies, which governments within Australia lacked. Almost all health workers were public servants or employees of missions subsidised by the state. The private practitioner was a very rare bird, except in the 1930s and since the 1970s. Secondly, the state in Papua New Guinea was usually an *Australian* state, accountable to the Commonwealth Government, staffed by Australian public servants according to Australian public service criteria and procedures. Through the Papua New Guinea administration, Australian interests could readily be expressed. What, then, were Australia's interests in the well-being of the inhabitants of the islands?

When Australia assumed responsibility for Papua early this century, the major concerns of the Commonwealth Governmnt were two: to secure British guarantees of defence support, and to achieve a 'white Australia' by excluding coloured immigrants, repatriating Pacific islanders, and isolating Aboriginal Australians. Fortress Australia as a strategic concept and white Australia as a social goal both implied the demobilisation of Melanesians and sufficient control over the arc of islands to inhibit their use in attacks on Australia. The strategy of quarantine and segregation was little more than the medical dimension of that social policy. The fact that medical arguments were used to justify quarantine and segregation should not obscure the strategic roots of that approach to public health.

The Great War confirmed Australians' identity as the white Gurkhas of the British Empire, sending volunteers to fight for the home country without asking awkward questions. Reliance on a volunteer army then created obligations towards the returned soldiers in peace time; and the reservation of public service positions in New Guinea and in Papua for ex-servicemen was a natural consequence. The further consequence – to enshrine military values as the operating principles of the New Guinea state – also flowed from the special status of ex-servicemen and their values. It is not difficult to see why the New Guinea administration between the wars (the only Australian state created from scratch after 1901) had a more militarist style than its Papuan counterpart, where significant numbers of pre-war staff were retained.

During the first, formative generation of this century, Australian authorities also sharpened their policies concerning race and gender. If Australia became (at least notionally) white, it also became 'a man's country'; and the colonial states across Torres Strait were white man's states. Two significant consequences flowed into health matters. First, the public role of expatriate women was subject to strict constraints: they could not be doctors in any circumstances, and as nurses they must minister only to white patients (in effect only to white men). The escape clause of this impossible equation was the mission service, staffed by women 'of the missionary type' who were subject to very different (and complementary) constraints on their behaviour. Secondly, medical authorities never managed to focus on women for more than the time required to write a single despatch. There was an unconscious but resonant harmony between Australian thinking and the frame of reference of the black men with whom Australian officers most commonly interacted. At no point before the 1940s did it strike medical authorities that there should be lots of nurses; nor did they consider that women's health issues might impinge upon the perceived depopulation of Melanesia. The virtues of the health services were partly vitiated by the large blind spots of medical planning – and in these blind spots Melanesian women lived and died.

The amalgamated Territory of Papua New Guinea after the Pacific War remained a 'man's country', in which gender roles laid down in the 1920s were slow to change. It also suffered a shortage of 'man-power' for economic production. The high infant mortality rate struck planners as destructive – and avoidable. And this *Australian* perception of a Papua New Guinea problem animated the new Division of Maternal and Child Welfare, the women's auxiliary of a department otherwise run by men, for men. Since women remained invisible in the public sphere, it was possible for a health strategy whose goal was a healthy and contented population, to ignore the ill-being of the female segment of that population.

By the 1960s Australian authorities recognised that their interests in Papua New Guinea would be best served by a contented and independent government. The creation of that independent government required more effective coordination of departmental activities than had been necessary during the high colonial era of the 1950s; so medical services were subordinated to some kind of bureaucratic review. Much of the restructuring of health policies and programmes in the 1960s had this end in view. At the end of Australian colonialism, as in the beginning, Australian social and strategic conceptions largely shaped the health services which evolved in Papua New Guinea. Even after Independence, Australian research priorities continue to influence the scope and direction of Papua New Guinea's medical research agenda.

We began by proposing that there were at least four ways of analysing the determinants of health policies and programmes. There is something to be said for all four kinds of analysis. Doctors have, in reality, dominated health policy-formation, and they have successfully resisted direct control by non-doctors. The medical profession and the Public Health Department have been thoroughly influenced by ideas and techniques which evolved elsewhere, through a nearly-universal medical profession. It is also true that the quality and quantity and general direction of health services have been constrained by the economic circumstances of the country itself, and by its ability to attract external funding. And Australian opinion has always and pervasively influenced Papua New Guinea medical services. In this context, there is little point in pursuing the argument further, to measure which form of argument best suits particular periods of medical history. We now know enough about the constraints on health policy, to suggest how it might be redirected.

We know, for instance, that any redirection must gain the support of at least a significant number of doctors. Their dominance over every other branch of the caring professions, and the deference which they enjoy from health workers, patients, and politicians ensures their ability to veto health policies and programmes which offend their professional judgement. The need to persuade doctors may seem to rule out any substantial change – until we remember that the medical profession has often shifted its perceptions and perspectives during the past hundred years, and that doctors are by no means monolithic in their judgements. The profession in Papua New Guinea is unusually attuned to public opinion: many doctors are first generation professionals, with lively social contacts outside the profession. Many others are motivated by an almost-missionary zeal to serve the general good; and opportunities for self-interested doctors are better in Australia than in Papua New Guinea. These circumstances help to explain the leadership of doctors (and especially doctors with a mission background) in the drive towards an integrated national service in the 1970s; and it was from doctors that the impulse came towards community involvement in policies and programmes. There is sufficient variety of opinion within the profession, to allow some room for manoeuvre.

Any shift in medical strategy would also require the sanction of at least some fraction of the world-wide profession: it is almost inconceivable that most doctors in Papua New Guinea would defy the accumulated wisdom of the World Health Organisation. Once again we may take comfort from the diversity of opinion within the profession at large. It was within the WHO that the shift towards primary health care was accomplished. That new perspective helped to validate a movement in the Medical Faculty of Papua New Guinea's University, away from the orthodoxy of Australian medical education in that era. Here again, there seems to be room for choice, albeit within strict limits.

Following the examples of Lambert and Gunther, medical reformers will need to analyse the political and economic realities of the country, and manipulate them to their purposes. Such skill does exist. In 1980 a coalition of public servants (mainly in the National Planning Office and the Department of Finance), politicians and doctors purged the Public Health Department of its centralists, and decentralised some functions to provincial authorities. Clearly then, medical policy is not frozen.

During the colonial era, Australian public opinion (and especially medical opinion) counted for much in Papua New Guinea. Since Independence, Australian public opinion weighs much less in the scales, but Australian medical interests can be significant. The decision to run a field trial for a new malaria vaccine in Papua New Guinea suggests that some programmes at least are designed to suit particular interests outside the country. Nevertheless, at least in principle Papua New Guinea public opinion could become significant as a source of policy and programmes. Thus far, that opinion has not expressed itself effectively in technical matters such as health: the shift of strategy in 1980, and the evolution of private practice since the 1970s, were the work of small and well-organised interest groups (such as public servants, teachers, and employees of the mining companies) and of the state itself. This is a substantial problem, since urbanised, salaried groups are much less at risk than the rest of the population, and are much the best served by a continuation of existing programmes. Health professionals and their programmes do respond to articulate public demand. How then, is it possible for the groups of people most at risk to exert as much influence as their urban wage-earning cousins on health programmes?

Our survey suggests that the people most at risk, and least able to gain access to services, include highland fringe-dwellers and rural women generally. How could women (for example) influence policy to their collective advantage? Here we must digress to ask how women in western societies have influenced the scope and nature of health services. On one front, western women have insisted that they should not be treated as an object during child-birth, but should retain dignity and control. By organising themselves, by gaining information, by winning the support of some obstetricians and midwives, they have placed the issue firmly on the medical agenda. There is also a powerful movement to regain control over their own reproduction, by fertility control, by de-criminalising abortion, and through the funding of free-standing women's health centres. Could rural women in Papua New Guinea wage such a campaign, despite their isolation from each other and from centres of power?

The essential first step would be the realisation that each woman's problem is not unique, but part of a national issue. Next they would need to phrase their demands (for ante-natal and post-natal care, among other services) in terms which would command wider attention. They might, for instance, argue that female mortality constitutes a national crisis, with consequences for social order, economic production, political stability and natural justice. Thirdly, they could insist upon a concerted approach by politicians, public servants, medical professionals and medical planners. In waging such a campaign, they would confront the tendency for medical services to be concentrated in urban areas, for health-givers to seek their own convenience, and for policy-makers to hear only the best organised lobbyists. By confronting these tendencies, they would be working for everyone's advantage.

Realistically, we cannot expect 'women' as a group, nor 'villagers' as a community, to leap fully-armed into public debate. Practical measures are now required to empower people to identify their health needs and to pursue them. These practical measures – public information in the form of public education programmes, and social information reintroduced to the professional training of medical workers – are entirely compatible with the strategy of primary health care. Of all the countries on earth, Papua New Guinea has the most vigorous tradition of parochial debate and local responsibility. If public health education could be harnessed to that parochial tradition, the effect would be powerfully therapeutic.

The doctors of the 1960s who argued for local participation and control were right then: and the argument is even stronger with the passage of time. In the 1960s there was a rough but creative tension between medical professionals and Australian public opinion. The removal of Australian lay opinion, through political independence, has upset that balance. Conversely, the rapid separation of urban, professional and salaried Papua New Guineans from their rural cousins leaves control over health programmes firmly in the hands of professionals and bureaucrats. Only the organisation and assertion of other elements of public opinion, can restore some vitality to the debate over medical issues. Without the creative impact of an organised public opinion, even the impressive services which the country now enjoys, must decline into a series of ritualised functions, whose original purpose recedes in the memory, which satisfies only the therapists, and which might even become (as in earlier days) the object of suspicion and superstition.

If the benefits of public participation are enormous, so are the costs of public indifference. Papua New Guinea's experience confirms that of many other modern societies: public health is mainly the outcome of the way people live, what they eat and drink, and how they work. The most glamorous medical interventions (which dramatically restore individual well-being) have the least impact on the health of the general public. Conversely, the greatest benefit is conferred by the least spectacular programmes. Left to their own devices, the medical profession might well be tempted towards technical sophistication. It is this health risk which requires the widest possible public participation in health affairs, so that the nation's health may be seen once again as a matter of universal concern, and is no longer a series of doctors' dilemmas.

Notes

1 Pre-colonial health and disease

1 Carol Jenkins, Editorial, 'The role of traditional medical practice in Papua New Guinea', *Papua New Guinea Medical Journal*, 27:3–4 (1984), 121.

2 See the three chapters by Jack Golson, in Donald Denoon and Catherine Snowden (eds.), *A history of agriculture in Papua New Guinea* (Port Moresby, 1981), pp. 33–42, 43–54, 55–64.

3 *Ibid*, pp. 33–42.

4 Ian Maddocks, 'Communicable diseases in Papua and New Guinea', in *PNGMedJ*, 13:4 (1970), 120. This is the text of Professor Maddocks' address to the ANZAAS Congress in Port Moresby in 1970.

5 J. Pernetta and L. Hill, 'Subsidy cycles in consumer/producer societies: the face of change', in Denoon and Snowden, *A history of agriculture in PNG*, pp. 293–309.

6 For the perils of small populations, see Norma MacArthur, 'Isolated populations in enclaves or on small islands', in R. J. May and Hank Nelson (eds.), *Melanesia: beyond diversity* (Canberra, 1982), I, pp. 27–32.

7 Golson, 'Agriculture in New Guinea: the long view', in Denoon and Snowden, *A history of agriculture in PNG*, pp. 33–42.

8 One such community is described by Albert Maori Kiki in his *Ten thousand years in a lifetime* (Melbourne, 1968).

9 See Jim Allen, 'Fishing for wallabies', in J. Friedman and M. J. Rowlands (eds.), *The evolution of social systems* (London, 1977) pp. 419–56: and Martha Macintyre, 'Changing paths: an historical ethnography of the traders of Tubetube', unpublished PhD thesis, Australian National University, 1983.

10 Ian Hughes, *New Guinea Stone Age trade* (Canberra, 1977).

11 Bryant Allen, personal communication, Canberra 1987 and N. N. Miklouho-Maclay, *Travels to New Guinea: diaries, letters, documents*, ed. D. Tumarkin (Moscow, 1982), Introduction.

12 This encounter is translated and published in J. K. Whittaker, N. G. Gash, J. F. Hookey and R. J. Lacey (eds.), *Documents and readings in New Guinea history: prehistory to 1889* (Brisbane, 1975), at p. 188.

13 See Miklouho-Maclay, *Travels to New Guinea*; and other contact experiences presented in Whittaker *et al.* (eds.), *Documents and readings*.

14 Ralph Garruto, 'Disease patterns of isolated groups', in Henry R. Rothschild (ed.), *Biocultural aspects of disease* (New York, 1981), p. 560.

15 Maddocks, 'Communicable diseases in Papua and New Guinea', p. 15.

16 Allen, 'Fishing for wallabies', pp. 435–8.

17 John Lourie, Tukutau Taufa, Jackie Cattani and Bill Anderson, 'Preliminary results of the Ok Tedi medical survey', paper presented at the 19th annual symposium of the Papua New Guinea Medical Society, Lae, September 1983.

18 Golson, 'Agriculture in New Guinea: the long view', pp. 33–42.

19 Garruto, 'Disease patterns of isolated groups', p. 561.
20 *Ibid*, pp. 561–3.
21 I am indebted to Stan Christian, practical malariologist par excellence, for the fruits of his 60 years' observations, Canberra 1985.
22 G. Crane, 'Perspectives on the treatment of Tropical Splenomegaly Syndrome', Proceedings of the 19th Annual Symposium of the PNG Medical Society, Lae, 1983.
23 John Stanhope, 'Patterns of fertility and mortality in rural New Guinea', *New Guinea Research Bulletin*, 34 (1970), 24–41.
24 Maddocks, 'Communicable diseases in Papua New Guinea', p. 120.
25 Garruto, 'Disease patterns of isolated groups' p. 577; and Dr Sue Serjeantson, personal communication.
26 Maddocks, 'Communicable disease in Papua New Guinea', p. 122.
27 Barry Shaw, 'The children of the Kyaka Enga', typescript, Development Studies Centre, Australian National University, 1981.
28 Dr J. Heydon, 'Observations in the mandated territory of New Guinea, December 1934 to February 1935', Australian Archives CRS, School of Public Health and Tropical Medicine; SP 1963/1, General Correspondence, 1930–1965, File 683, held at Australian Archives, Sydney.
29 Maddocks, 'Communicable diseases in Papua New Guinea', p. 122.
30 Bryant Allen, personal communication, Canberra 1987.
31 Stan Wigley, 'Tuberculosis and New Guinea: historical perspectives with special reference to the years from 1871 to 1973', in B. G. Burton-Bradley (ed.), *The history of medicine in Papua New Guinea* (Sydney, in press).
32 B. M. du Toit, *Akuna: a New Guinea village community* (Rotterdam, 1975), p. 152.
33 H. R. Parkinson, *Dreissig Jahre in der Südsee* (Stuttgart, 1907).
34 Dr Timothy Pyakalyia, interviewed by Dr Leslie Marshall, Medical History Tapes (hereinafter MHR) No 20, held in University of Papua New Guinea Library (New Guinea Collection) and the Reading Room of the Department of Pacific and Southeast Asian History, Australian National University.
35 du Toit, *Akuna*, p. 153.
36 Borut Telban, personal communication, Port Moresby 1987.
37 F. B. Smith, *The people's health 1830–1910* (Canberra, 1979).
38 William E. Mitchell, 'Culturally contrasting therapeutic systems of the West Sepik: the Lujere', in T. R. Williams (ed.), *Psychological anthropology* (The Hague, 1975), p. 435.
39 M. P. Alpers, D. C. Gajdusek and S. G. Ono, *Bibliography of Kuru* (Bethesda, 1975); and J. T. Gunther, 'Kuru and a Nobel Prize', mimeo, Department of Pacific & Southeast Asian History, Australian National University.
40 R. W. Hornabrook (ed.), *Essays on Kuru* (Faringdon, 1976) provides an excellent introduction to the subject.
41 For example, R. Fleming Jones, 'Tropical diseases in British New Guinea', *Transactions of the Royal Society for Tropical Medical Hygiene*, v (1910–11) 93–105; and William MacGregor, 'Some problems of tropical medicine', *Lancet*, 13 October 1900, pp. 1055–61.
42 Staniforth Smith (presumably on the advice of Dr W. M Strong, the Government Medical Officer in Papua), *Handbook of the Territory of Papua* (3rd edn, Melbourne, 1912), p. 19.
43 Garruto, 'Disease patterns of isolated groups', pp. 579–80.
44 Fleming Jones, 'Tropical diseases in British New Guinea'.
45 Stanhope, 'Patterns of fertility and mortality', p. 36.

46 These patterns of behaviour are described in Gilbert Herdt (ed.), *Ritualized* homosexuality in Melanesia (Berkeley and London, 1984); and considered by Maddocks in 'Communicable diseases in Papua New Guinea'.

47 B. S. Hetzel and P. O. D. Pharoah (eds.), *Endemic cretinism* (Goroka, 1971), pp. 5–8.

48 Heydon, 'Observations in the Mandated Territory', see note 28 above.

49 Carol Jenkins, 'Indigenous childbirth practices', *PNGMedJ*, xxvii, 2 (1984), pp. 61–4.

50 The estimates are collected by David A. M. Lea and Laurie H. Lewis, 'Masculinity in Papua New Guinea', in L. A. Kosinski and J. W. Webb (eds.), *Population at Microscale* (New Zealand Geographical Society, Auckland, 1976), pp. 65–78.

51 Patricia K. Townsend, 'Infant mortality in the Saniyo-Hiyowe population, Ambunti District, East Sepik Province', *PNGMedJ*, 28:3 (1985), 177–82.

52 Lea and Lewis, 'Masculinity in Papua New Guinea' pp. 65–78; and D. J. van de Kaa 'The demography of Papua New Guinea's indigenous population', unpublished PhD thesis, Australian National University, 1971.

53 This point is made by several nutrition and MCH workers interviewed in the MHR series, e.g. Holzknechts (3 and 4), Crouch (5, 6 and 7), Smith (16), Tinsley Health Workers (17 and 18), and Deaseys (22 and 23).

54 A clear account is given by Robert M. May, 'Parasitic infections as regulators of animal populations', *American Scientist*, 71 (1983), 36–45.

2 The administration of public health

1 L. Doyal with I. Pennell, *The political economy of health* (London, 1979), chapter 7, 'Medicine and imperialism'.

2 Smith, *The people's health*, pp. 415ff.

3 The following paragraphs rely heavily on T. S. Pensabene, *The rise of the medical practitioner in Victoria* (Canberra, 1980), and Evan Willis, *Medical dominance: the division of labour in Australian health care* (Sydney, 1983).

4 C. J. Cummins, *A history of medical administration in New South Wales, 1788–1973* (Sydney, 1979), p. 63.

5 Philip D. Curtin, 'Medical knowledge and urban planning in tropical Africa', in *American Historical Review*, 90:3 (1985), 594–613, p. 594.

6 Roger Joyce, *Sir William MacGregor* (Melbourne, 1971), pp. 1–11.

7 Fleming Jones, 'Tropical diseases in British New Guinea', pp. 93–4.

8 Michael Worboys, 'The emergence of tropical medicine: a study in the establishment of a scientific speciality', in G. LeMaine, R. MacLeod *et el*. (eds.), *Perspectives on the emergence of scientific disciplines* (The Hague, 1976), pp. 75–98, esp. pp. 80–81.

9 *Ibid.*, pp. 88–93.

10 Joyce, *MacGregor*, pp. 219–39.

11 Curtin, 'Medical knowledge and urban planning in Africa', *passim*.

12 Maynard W. Swanson, 'The sanitation syndrome: bubonic plague and urban native policy in the Cape Colony, 1900–1909', *Journal of African History*, 18:3, (1977), 387–410.

13 R. A. Douglas, 'Dr Anton Breinl and the Australian Institute of Tropical Medicine', *MJA*, 1 (1977), pp. 713–16. See also Lyn Harloe, 'Anton Breinl and the Australian Institute of Tropical Medicine', ANZAAS Congress paper, Townsville, 1987.

14 See for example A. Grenfell Price, 'The white man in the tropics', *MJA*, 1 (1935), pp. 106–10.
15 Sir Raphael Cilento, in R. W. Cilento and C. Lack, *Triumph in the tropics: an historical sketch of Queensland* (Brisbane, 1959), p. 426.
16 AITM Circular Letter, signed by Cilento, 30 November 1922, in Australian Archives, CRS, Sydney: School of Public Health and Tropical Medicine series, SP 106/1, General Correspondence 1908–1955, file 65.
17 Joyce, *MacGregor*, pp. 229–36.
18 Sir William MacGregor, 'Some problems of tropical medicine', *Lancet*, 13 October 1900, pp. 1055–61.
19 William H. Ewers, 'Malaria in the early years of German New Guinea', *Journal of the Papua New Guinea Society*, 6 (1973), 1.
20 Fleming Jones, 'Tropical diseases in British New Guinea', p. 93.
21 Douglas, 'Breinl and the AITM', p. 750.
22 Circular correspondence in CAO, CP 78/20; and in CRS A518, 832/1/1.
23 e.g. CRS: A 518, D 832/1/3. Correspondence concerning the First International Pacific Health Conference in Melbourne, 1925 and 1926.
24 CRS Sydney, archives of the School of Public Health and Tropical Medicine, CS 1061, box 17, item 449. Cilento's memo for file, 30 June 1929.
25 *Ibid*, S. P. 1061, box 79, item 635, Dr Harvey Sutton's correspondence with Advisory Board of the Racial Hygiene Association of New South Wales during the 1930s.
26 Quoted in Worboys, 'The emergence of tropical medicine', p. 85.
27 Curtin, 'Medical knowledge and urban planning in Africa', *passim*.
28 Donald Denoon, 'Temperate medicine and settler capitalism: on the reception of western medical ideas', in R. MacLeod (ed.), *Disease, medicine and empire* (Routledge, London, in press), pp. 124–5.

3 Early colonial medical administration

1 Miklouho-Maclay, *Travels to New Guinea*, p. 13.
2 S. Latukefu, 'Oral history and Pacific Island missionaries', in D. Denoon and R. Lacey (eds.), *Oral tradition in Melanesia* (Port Moresby, 1981), pp. 182–3.
3 Hank Nelson, *Black, white and gold: goldmining in Papua New Guinea, 1878–1930* (Canberra, 1976), pp. 192–205.
4 Papers of John Cameron, held in Department of Pacific and Southeast Asian History, Australian National University, letter dated 1889.
5 Curtin, 'Medical knowledge and urban planning', *passim*.
6 *Ibid*, p. 595.
7 Ewers, 'Malaria in the early years of German New Guinea', p. 9. Ewers's quotation from Dr Schellong comes from O. Schellong, 'Die Neu-Guinea-Malaria einst und jetzt', *Archiv für Schiffs-und Tropen-Hygiene*, 5 (1901).
8 *Ibid*, pp. 9–12.
9 Fleming Jones, 'Tropical diseases in British New Guinea', p. 97.
10 The condition of an infected population is taken from the description by A. Balfour and H. H. Scott, *Health problems of the empire: past, present and future* (London, 1924), cited in Ewers, p. 3.
11 The German New Guinea Annual Reports have been translated and edited by P. Sack and D. Clark (Canberra, 1979) and are cited as GNGAR, in this instance 1889–90.
12 Stewart Firth, *New Guinea under the Germans* (Melbourne, 1983) pp. 171–2; Peter Sack, 'A history of German New Guinea: a debate about evidence and

judgement', *JPH*, 20:1–2 (1985) 84–94; and Stewart Firth, 'German New Guinea: the archival perspective', in the same edition of JPH, pp. 94–103.
13 GNGAR, 1892–93.
14 *Ibid.*
15 Firth, *New Guinea under the Germans*, pp. 161–74.
16 British New Guinea Annual Reports (hereinafter BNGAR), 1886.
17 *Ibid*, to 1906. The incumbents are also listed in Ellen Kettle, *That they might live* (Sydney, 1979).
18 Donald Denoon, 'Walter Mersh Strong', in B. G. Burton-Bradley (ed.), *The history of medicine in PNG* (Sydney, in press).
19 Robert Black, 'Dr. Bellamy of Papua', three-part article, in *MJA*, 2 (1957), pp. 189–97, 232–8, 279–84.
20 Kettle, *That they might live*, p. 14.
21 Sir John Gunther's obituary in *PNGMedJ*, 1:2 (1955), 81.
22 S. M. Lambert, *Doctor in paradise* (London, 1942), p. 19.
23 Papuan Annual Report (hereinafter PAR), 1920.
24 CRS, A. 518, U.832/1/5. Murray to Minister, 2 November 1938.
25 Kettle, *That they might live*, pp. 12–13; PAR, 1909.
26 GNGAR, 1889–90.
27 Charles Rowley, 'The promotion of native health in German New Guinea', *South Pacific*, 9:5 (1957), 396–9.
28 Neville Hicks, *'This sin and scandal': Australia's population debate, 1891–1911* (Canberra, 1978); and Pensabene, *The rise of the medical practitioner*, pp. 24–6.
29 Doyal with Pennell, 'Medicine and imperialism', pp. 239–90.
30 Curtin, 'Medical knowledge and urban planning', p. 613.
31 Denoon, 'Strong'; Black, 'Bellamy', pp. 12–16.
32 Strong, in Staniforth Smith (ed.), *Handbook for the Territory of Papua*, p. 18.
33 S. S. MacKenzie, *The Australians at Rabaul* (4th edn, Sydney, 1937), p. 81.
34 A. G. Butler *et al.*, *The Australian Army Medical Services in the War of 1914–1918* (2nd edn, Melbourne, 1938), p. 790.
35 *Ibid*, pp. 794–6.
36 *Ibid*, pp. 796–7.
37 *Ibid*, pp. 801–2.
38 Mackenzie, *Australians at Rabaul*, p. 218.
39 *Ibid*, p. 365.
40 Ian Maddocks, 'Communicable disease in Papua New Guinea', pp. 120–1.
41 MacGregor, 'Problems of tropical medicine' pp. 1055–61; Nelson, *Black, white and gold*, pp. 192–231.
42 Quoted in Firth, *New Guinea under the Germans*, p. 113.
43 Ian Maddocks, 'Medicine and colonialism', *Australian and New Zealand Journal of Sociology*, 11:3 (1975), 29.
44 Black, 'Bellamy', *passim*.
45 Wigley, 'Tuberculosis in New Guinea'.
46 Heydon, 'Observations in the mandated territory of New Guinea'; and F. W. Clements, 'A tuberculosis survey of a Papuan village', *MJA*, 2 (1936), pp. 253–8.
47 Clements, quoted in C. R. Hallpike, *Bloodshed and vengeance in the Papuan mountains: the generation of conflict in Tauade society* (Oxford, 1977), p. 49.
48 R. Cilento, *The causes of the depopulation of the western islands of the territory of New Guinea* (Canberra, 1928).
49 Fleming Jones, 'Tropical diseases in British New Guinea', p. 96.

4 The political economy of health in Papua between the wars
1 John Mayo, 'Oddity of empire: British New Guinea 1884–88', unpublished MA thesis, University of Papua New Guinea, 1972. For a broader discussion, see J. T. Griffin, Hank Nelson and S. G. Firth, *Papua New Guinea: a political history* (Melbourne, 1979).
2 PAR, 1927/28 to 1935/36.
3 Griffin, Nelson and Firth, *Political history*, pp. 25–6.
4 *Ibid*, pp. 27–8.
5 PAR, 1933/34.
6 Personal communication, Sydney, 1982.
7 Robert Black, 'Bellamy of Papua', *passim*; and CRS, A518–832/1/5. Cumpston to Department of Territories, 15 May 1935.
8 Francis West (ed.), *Selected letters of Hubert Murray* (Melbourne, 1970), Hubert Murray to Atlee Hunt, 18 August 1913.
9 PAR, 1928/29 and 1933/34.
10 *Ibid*, 1935/36.
11 W. H. Wallace, *The Wallace story* (Melbourne, n.d. (?1972)), p. 44. Dr Wallace held an acting appointment in Port Moresby in 1926.
12 CRS, A 518, S 832/1/5, correspondence with Dr Alec May and the Misima mine management, 1937/38.
13 Critical judgments in Lambert, *A doctor in paradise*, pp. 19ff, and Wallace, *The Wallace story*, pp. 44–5.
14 CRS, A 1928: 775/11. Strong to Commonwealth Director-General of Health, 21 May 1937.
15 H. N. Nelson, 'Brown doctors, white prejudice', *New Guinea*, 5:2 (1970), pp. 21–8.
16 PAR, 1926/27. MHA Tape 11, interview with Hera Ganiga, Port Moresby 1981, by Fr Leo Wearden.
17 Walter Mersh Strong, 'The medical education of Papuan natives', *MJA*, 2 (1935), pp. 305–9, cited and discussed in Ian Maddocks, 'Medicine and colonialism', pp. 30–33.
18 Interview with Sir John Gunther, Melbourne 1982; and interview with Stan Christian, Canberra 1982.
19 Lambert, *Doctor in paradise*, p. 19.
20 Price, 'White man in the tropics', pp. 106–10.
21 In Staniforth Smith (ed.), *Handbook*, p. 18.
22 Walter Mersh Strong, 'Nutritional aspects of depopulation and disease in the western Pacific, especially in Papua', *MJA*, 2 (1932), pp. 506–12.
23 On Rockefeller generally, see Victor Heiser, *A Doctor's Odyssey: adventures in forty-five countries* (London, 1936); and on Papua New Guinea, see Lambert, *Doctor in paradise*.
24 Lambert, *Doctor in paradise*, p. 99.
25 Strong, *Bacillary dysentery* (Port Moresby, 1932); *The feeding of native labourers in Papua* (Port Moresby, 1926); and *Improving the food supplies of native villages* (Port Moresby 1926).
26 Lambert, *Doctor in paradise*, pp. 28ff.
27 CRS, CS 1061, Box 16, file 408. J. B. Clark to Administrator Staniforth Smith, 20 February 1922.
28 *Ibid*, Smith to Minister, 22 February 1922.
29 *Ibid*, Box 17, file 440, Strong's memo of 30 June 1926.
30 Interviews with Gunther, Melbourne 1982, and Christian, Canberra, 1982.

31 PAR, 1925/6.
32 CRS A1929, 775/12 (Department of Health), 'Papua – establishment at Gemo of Hospital for treatment of leprosy and tuberculosis'; Gemo Island Hospital Report by Constance Fairhall, November 1938.
33 Interview with Keke Maleva, Port Moresby, 1981.
34 Amirah Inglis, *Karo: the life and fate of a Papuan* (Canberra, 1982), pp. 61–70.
35 Dr Joan Refshauge's Papers, Australian National Library. Dr Refshauge describes the conditions she inherited on moving to Papua in 1946.
36 Michael Young, 'A tropology of the Dobu Mission', *Canberra Anthropology*, 3 (1980) 86–104; and his 'Suffer the children: Wesleyans in the D'Entrecasteaux', in Margaret Jolly and Martha Macintyre (eds.), *Family and gender in the Pacific: domestic contradictions and the colonial impact* (Cambridge, 1988).
37 D. Langmore, 'European missionaries in Papua 1984–1914, a group portrait', Unpublished PhD thesis, Australian National University 1981.
38 Young, 'Suffer the children'.
39 Young, 'A tropology of the Dobu Mission', pp. 97–100.
40 For information on English university medical curricula in the nineteenth century, I am indebted to Dr F. B. Smith.
41 PAR, 1921/2.
42 CRS, A 518, Item N 840/1/5. Strong's memo dated 16 July 1930, enclosed in Murray to Minister, 6 September 1930.
43 *Ibid*, Murray to Minister, 5 January 1931.
44 *Ibid*, Murray to Minister, 30 January 1935, enclosing report by Mrs A Wiles, Infant Welfare Nurse for the SDA mission.
45 Berkeley Vaughan, *Doctor in Papua* (Adelaide, 1974) pp. 40–57. See also, MHR tapes of interviews with Cecil Abel (10) and Nedulia (9).
46 *Ibid*, MHR tapes 22 and 23.
47 In the reports listed at notes 41 and 42 above.
48 Kettle, *That they might live*; and MHR tapes 3, 4, 5, 6, 7, 9, 10.
49 CRS A 1928: 775/9. Frank Molomy to Director CSIRO, 10 August 1940; and Cumpston's reply, 20 August 1940.
50 CRS, A 1928: 775/6. H. Sutton (Director of the School) to Director-General of Health, Canberra, 18 July 1935, quoting a letter from Dr A. Heaslip.
51 I discuss the nature of Australian colonialism in 'Capitalism in Papua New Guinea', *JPH*, 20:3–4 (1985), 119–34.
52 R. F. R. Scragg, 'Lemankoa, 1920–1980: a study of the effects of health care interventions' unpublished MA thesis, University of Sydney, 1983.

5 The political economy of health in New Guinea between the wars

1 James Gillespie, 'The hookworm campaign and a national health policy in Australia, 1911–1930', ANZAAS Congress paper Townsville 1987; and Margaret Spencer, *John Howard Lidgett Cumpston 1880–1954* (privately published, Tenterfield NSW, 1987), pp. 98–103.
2 Spencer, *Cumpston*, pp. 186–91; R. W. Cilento, 'Obituary: J. S. C. Elkington', *MJA*, 1 (1955) pp. 144–5; D. Gordon, 'Obituary: Sir Raphael West Cilento', *MJA*, 1 (1985) pp. 259–60; and J. H. L. Cumpston, *Health and disease in Australia* (ed. Milton Lewis, in preparation for publication), Lewis's Introduction.
3 Spencer, *Cumpston*, p. 227; Lewis's Introduction to Cumpston, *Health and disease in Australia*.
4 Gillespie, 'The hookworm campaign and a national health policy'; Spencer, *Cumpston*, pp. 250–4.

5 Spencer, *Cumpston*, pp. 227ff; Lewis's Introduction to Cumpston, *Health and disease in Australia*.

6 P. Hernant and R. W. Cilento, *Report of the mission entrusted with a survey on health conditions in the Pacific Islands* (League of Nations Health Organisation, Geneva, 1929).

7 *Pacific Islands Monthly*, 4 (January 1934), p. 27.

8 CRS, A 518, A 832/1/5. Murray (on leave in Switzerland) to High Commissioner in London, 14 December 1928.

9 On the Expropriation Board, see Patricia Hopper, 'Kicking out the Hun', Unpublished MA thesis, University of Papua New Guinea, 1980.

10 Butler, *Australian Army Medical Services*, pp. 799–800.

11 Lambert, *Doctor in paradise*, p. 77.

12 CRS, A 518, F 832/1/3. Cilento to Minister, January 1925; and A 457:741/1 Administrator to Prime Minister, 15 February 1922.

13 Hopper, 'Kicking out the Hun'.

14 Cilento, *White man in the tropics*, p. 95.

15 Cited in Ian Maddocks Editorial, *PNGMedJ*, 10:2 (June 1967), 33–4, quoting the Standing Orders for the Department of Public Health, 1924.

16 Cilento, *White man in the tropics*, p. 168.

17 New Guinea Annual Report to the League of Nations (hereinafter NGAR), 1925–26.

18 *Ibid*, 1924–25.

19 Personal communication, Stan Christian, Canberra, 1982.

20 For an account of Lucas, see Buckley and Klugman, *Burns Philp*.

21 CRS, A 518, R 832/1/3. Lucas to Prime Minister's Secretary, 21 July 1922.

22 *Ibid*, 15 August 1922.

23 *Ibid*, memo from Director of Public Health, August 1922.

24 Hopper, 'Kicking out the Hun'.

25 CRS, A 518, F 832/1/3. Cilento to Minister, January 1925.

26 NGAR throughout the 1920s and 1930s.

27 Interview, Stan Christian, Canberra, 1982.

28 CRS, A 518, 0 832/1/3. New Guinea estimates for 1922/23, enclosing report from Dr J. H. S. Jackson, Medical Officer at Kavieng.

29 NGAR 1938–39; and interview with Stan Christian.

30 Robin Radford, *Highlanders and foreigners in the Upper Ramu: the Kainantu Area 1919–1942* (Melbourne, 1987), pp. 40–60.

31 CRS, A 518: F852/1/4, correspondence regarding recruitment of medical staff, 1921 onwards.

32 e.g. Heydon's report, 1935, cited in Chapter 1, fn 28.

33 Sir John Gunther, interview, Melbourne, 1982, records visiting the islands where Cilento conducted his demographic research, and being informed that Cilento stayed only for one night.

34 NGAR, 1921/22.

35 CRS, A 518, G 852/1/4. Part II. Deputy Administrator Wanliss to Prime Minister's Secretary, 4 October 1930.

36 Wigley, 'Tuberculosis in New Guinea'; and R. Scragg, 'Depopulation in New Ireland: a study of demography and fertility' unpublished MD thesis, University of Adelaide, 1954.

37 NGAR, 1925/26.

38 *Ibid*, 1938/39.

39 Cilento, 'Nutrition and numbers', *The Livingstone lectures, 1936*.

40 CRS, A 518, U 832/1/3, unsigned and undated memo, attributed to Cilento by context and internal evidence.
41 CRS, A 518, G 852/1/4, part III. Director-General Cumpston to Prime Minister's Secretary, 27 April 1939, and again 4 July 1940.
42 Refshauge reminiscences.
43 The subjects on which Senior Medical Assistants were tested, are given in NGAR, 1921–22. See also Christian interview.
44 NGAR, 1927–28.
45 Kettle, *That they might live*, pp. 98–116.
46 NGAR, 1926/7.

6 Medical education

1 See Chapter 4.
2 Port Moresby, 1917.
3 C. D. Rowley, 'The promotion of native health in German New Guinea', pp. 392–3.
4 Klaus Neumann, 'Will the missionary shoot the "smallpox spirit"' seminar paper, Pacific History, Australian National University, 1985.
5 NGAR, 1921–22.
6 *Ibid*, 1938–39.
7 Personal communication, Stan Christian.
8 *Ibid*.
9 CRS, A 518: H 852/1/4, correspondence 1922–24.
10 Walter Mersh Strong, 'The medical education of Papuan natives', *MJA*, 1 (1933), pp. 305–9.
11 CRS, A 518, U 832/1/3. Extract from Lambert to Brennan, 7 December 1932.
12 *Ibid*, Brennan's memo of 9 September 1932.
13 *Ibid*, Cumpston's memo of 30 November 1932.
14 *Ibid*, unsigned and undated memo, attributed to Cilento by context and internal evidence.
15 *Ibid*, Griffith to Minister, 25 November 1932.
16 Editorial, *Pacific Islands Monthly*, 7 (December 1936).
17 Strong, 'Medical education of Papuan natives', *passim*.
18 CRS, A 518 U 832/1/3; W. M. Strong (in Sydney) to Secretary, Prime Minister's Department, 27 November 1933.
19 *Ibid*; and *Wantok*, 31 January 1981, '47 Yia Bihain'.
20 Hank Nelson, 'Brown doctors, white prejudice', pp. 21–8.
21 Personal communication, John Gunther.
22 In Chapter 4.
23 See note 14.

7 The Pacific War

1 The standard works on medical conditions during the war are the four volumes in Series 5 (Medical) of *Australia in the War of 1939–1945*: Allan S. Walker, *Clinical problems of war* (Canberra, 1952); Walker, *Middle East and Far East* (Canberra, 1953); Walker, *The island campaigns* (Canberra, 1957); and A. S. Walker *et al.*, *Medical Services of the RAN and RAAF* (Canberra, 1961). The account of pre-war medical preparations is from these volumes, and in an interview with Sir William Refshauge, Canberra, 1982.

2 Walker, *The island campaigns*, pp. 1–14; and Gavin Long, *The final campaigns*, in Series 1 (Army) of the same project (Canberra, 1963), pp. 1–30.
3 Refshauge, interview.
4 Walker, *The island campaigns*, p. 123.
5 Refshauge, interview.
6 Walker, *The island campaigns*, p 72.
7 Long, *The final campaigns*, p. 237.
8 Hank Nelson, 'A note on the scale of the dying: the Japanese, 1942–1945', in R. J. May and Hank Nelson, (eds.) *Melanesia: beyond diversity* (Canberra, 1982), I, pp. 175–8.
9 MacKenzie, *Australians at Rabaul*, p. 365.
10 Private Papers, Brigadier H. C. Disher, held in Melbourne University Archives.
11 Walker, *The island campaigns*, p. 116.
12 *Ibid*, pp. 363–6 and Refshauge, interview.
13 Refshauge, interview.
14 *Ibid*; Gunther, interview; Walker, *The island campaigns*, pp. 364–6.
15 Walker, *The island campaigns* pp. 240–3; Gunther, interview.
16 Refshauge, interview.
17 Long, *The final campaigns*, Appendix 7.
18 Neville Robinson, *Villagers at war: some Papua New Guinea experiences in World War II* (Canberra, 1979), pp. 14–42.
19 Catherine Snowden, 'Copra co-operatives', in Denoon and Snowden, *A History of agriculture in PNG*, pp. 185–204.
20 Alan Leadley, 'Effects of Japanese occupation on Tolai people', Unpublished MA thesis, University of Papua New Guinea, 1973.
21 Cilento, 'Nutrition and numbers', pp. 35–6.
22 CRS, A 518, EO 840/1/4, part 1. Report of New Guinea Native Labour Commission, 1939.
23 Christian, interview.
24 CRS, A 518, EO 840/1/4, part 1. Minute by R. Melrose, 22 May 1945.
25 *Ibid*; Minister for the Army to Minister for Territories, 18 December 1945.
26 Joan Refshauge, interviewed by her brother.
27 John Burton, 'A dysentery epidemic in New Guinea, and its mortality', *JPH*, 18: 4 (1983) 236–61. See also Bryant Allen, 'A bomb or a bullet or the bloody flux', *ibid*, 218–35.
28 Kettle, *That they might live*, pp. 74–97.
29 MHR Tape 15, interview with Siming Aksim.
30 e.g. cases cited by Cecil Abel, MHR Tape 10; and Christian, interview.
31 Brian Jinks, 'Policy, planning and administration in Papua New Guinea, 1942–1952, with special reference to the role of Colonel J. K. Murray (Unpublished PhD thesis, University of Sydney, 1975), pp. 106–7.
32 For example MHR. Tapes 12 to 15, in which Ed Tscharke describes his own training on Gemo Island near Port Moresby.
33 Prologue, xxi.
34 S. A. Waksman, *The conquest of tuberculosis* (Berkeley and Los Angeles, 1966), pp. 119–46.
35 Refshauge, interview.
36 Scragg, 'Lemankoa', p. 32.

8 Miracle drugs, new perceptions

1 MHR Tape 10.
2 Interview with Sir John Gunther.
3 John Burton, 'A dysentery epidemic in New Guinea, and its mortality', p. 239.
4 Interview with Sir John Gunther.
5 Waksman, *The conquest of tuberculosis*, pp. 119ff.
6 See Chapter 3 above.
7 Robert H. Black, 'Health education in Papua and New Guinea', *South Pacific*, 10:1 (1958), 1–7. Originally given as a lecture at the Australian school of Pacific Administration in Sydney.
8 Brian Jinks, 'Australia's post-war policy for New Guinea and Papua', *JPH*, 17: 1–2 (1982), 86–100.
9 The quantities of money are set out in Denoon, 'Capitalism in Papua New Guinea', p. 125.
10 *Ibid.*
11 CRS, A 518 B 927/1, correspondence and memorandum early 1950, drafting a letter (undated on this file) from R. Halligan, the Secretary of the Department, to Administrator J. K. Murray. Included in the correspondence is this statement, attributed to John Crawford, at that time Secretary of the Department of Commerce.
12 *Ibid.*
13 CRS, A 1928. 710/26. Director-General McCallum to PMO Repatriation Commission Brisbane, 22 September 1945.
14 *Ibid*, McCallum's memo of 26 September 1945.
15 Jinks, 'Policy, planning and J. K. Murray', pp. 347–8.
16 Gunther, interview.
17 Doctors Deland and May survived the war, but did not hold policy-making positions, either before or after.
18 Gunther, interview.
19 *Ibid.* Brennan served on a committee to advise on post-war hospital construction, which reported in favour of Gunther's substantial programme.
20 Jinks, 'Australia's post-war policy' reports the criticism, pp. 97–100; the expenditure over time is tabulated by Gunther, 'Medical services, history', in *Encyclopaedia of Papua New Guinea*.
21 Jinks, 'Australia's post-war policy'.
22 Stan Christian, interview.
23 Jinks, 'Australia's post-war policy'.
24 J. T. Gunther, 'A report on the present position of the Department of Public Health', appendix E of a general progress report by the Administrator in 1950, in CRS, A 518, H 927/1. The rubbery quality of the report lies in its counting of segregated pre-war hospitals as a single institution, when two were located in the same place.
25 This situation prevailed until the 1950s, and is treated in Gunther's interview and his interview with E. F. Kunz; and in E. F. Kunz, *The intruders: refugee doctors in Australia* (Canberra, 1975), pp. 52–9.
26 Gunther, 'Report on the present position'.
27 Gunther, interview; and Joan Rafshauge's interview with her brother.
28 Draft advertisement, enclosed in Department of Territories memo of 16 January 1951, in CRS, A 518, B 852/6/3, part 2.
29 *Ibid*, part 1.
30 *Ibid*, part 2.

31 *Ibid*, part 1; Gunther to Halligan, 23 November 1946. See also Gunther, 'The present position'.
32 *Ibid* and interview.
33 CRS, A 1928, 710/26, correspondence dated 18 March 1946.
34 Refshauge, interview with her brother.
35 Gunther, interview.
36 Kettle, *That they might live*, attributes that break-through to the directorship of Dr Roy Scragg, p. 100.
37 Kunz, *The intruders*, pp. 52–9; Charles Haszler, 'The new Australian Doctors in New Guinea', *PNGMedJ*, 10:2 (1967), 35–42.
38 The relevant departmental circular is kept in Dr Joan Refshauge's papers, in the National Library of Australia, Canberra.
39 Sir William Refshauge, interview.
40 Christian, interview.
41 Gunther, interview.
42 *Ibid*.
43 Anthony J. Radford, 'Papua New Guinea's barefoot doctors, the aid post orderly and his predecessor the medical tultul', in H. Attwood and R. W. Home (eds.), *Patients, practitioners and techniques* (Melbourne, 1984), pp. 115–27.

9 The health campaigns

1 Gunther, interviews.
2 *Ibid*.
3 Described by J. A. Logan, The Sardinian Project (Baltimore, 1953) and summarised by Black, 'Health education'.
4 A. D. Parkinson and N. W. Tavil, 'Malaria', in Clive Bell (ed.) *The diseases and health services of Papua New Guinea* (Port Moresby, 1973), pp. 162–78.
5 Christian, interviews. The idea of complete eradication from particular areas was revived by W. Peters, 'Malaria control in Papua New Guinea', *PNGMedJ*, 3:3 (1959), 66–75.
6 J. T. Gunther, Epidemiology of Malaria in Papua New Guinea', *PNGMedJ*, I, 1 (1955) 1. This is the text of an address first given in a post-graduate lecture in Port Moresby, 20 July 1954.
7 Parkinson and Tavil, 'Malaria', pp. 162–78.
8 *Ibid*.
9 J. D. Charlwood, 'Which way now for Malaria control?', *PNGMedJ*, 28:3–4 (1984), 159–62.
10 Peter Sharp and Philip Harvey, 'Malaria and growth stunting in young children of the highlands of Papua New Guinea', *PNGMedJ*, 23:3 (1980), 132–40.
11 e.g. Charlwood, 'Which way now for Malaria control?', pp. 159–62.
12 This reference (like much of the following paragraphs) relies on S. C. Wigley, 'Tuberculosis and New Guinea: historical perspectives'.
13 *Ibid*.
14 *Ibid*, and Joan Refshauge, interview, and E. Fairhall, 'Report'.
15 Waksman, *The conquest of tuberculosis*, pp. 119ff.
16 CRS, A 518; P 832/1/6. Gunther to Halligan, 6 October 1949; and Gunther to Administrator, 14 November 1950.
17 *Ibid*, memo by Dr H. Wunderly, 19 November 1951, and Gunter's reply, 13 December 1951.
18 Wigley, 'Tuberculosis and New Guinea'.
19 Wigley, 'Tuberculosis', in Bell, *Diseases and health services*, pp. 179–84.

20 *Ibid.*
21 Refshauge, interview.
22 D. A. Russell and C. O. Bell, 'Leprosy', in Bell, *Diseases and health services*, pp. 185–90.
23 *Ibid.*
24 S. G. Browne, 'Prospects for the control of leprosy in Papua New Guinea', *PNGMedJ*, 26:1 (1983), 1–2.
25 Black, 'Health education', p. 1–7.
26 Charlwood, 'Which way now for Malaria control?' pp. 159–62.
27 Department of Health and National Planning Office, *1983 Health Policy Review* (Port Moresby, 1986), p. 2.
28 E. H. Hipsley and F. W. Clements (eds.), *Report of the New Guinea Nutrition Survey Expedition, 1947* (Department of External Territories, Canberra, 1947).
29 Gunther, interview.

10 Women and children last

1 Edwin G. Tscharke, *A quarter century of healing* (Madang, 1973), *passim*.
2 Gunther is quoted in the editorial of the *PNGMedJ* 9:4 (1966), 117–18. See also J. Nash, 'The role of the Leprosy Mission in the national tuberculosis/leprosy programme', Papua New Guinea Medical Society 19th Annual Symposium, Lae 1983.
3 Michael Young, 'A tropology of the Dobu Mission', pp. 97–100.
4 CRS, A518, R 832/1/6. Murray to Minister, 24 September 1949.
5 *Ibid*, Murray to Kendall, 31 January 1950. By this time, Gunther thought that the national infant mortality rate was above 250 per thousand but below 500.
6 Refshauge Papers, Australian National Library. Quotation from the text of an address to a women's organisation (possibly The Australian Federation of Business and Professional Women) in Brisbane after leaving Papua New Guinea.
7 *Ibid.* Transcript of interview with her brother William.
8 *Ibid*, draft Annual Reports of the division of Maternal and Child Health. See also Kettle, *That they might live*, pp. 101–2.
9 *Ibid*, draft Annual Report for 1952/53.
10 *Ibid*, draft Annual Report for 1953/54.
11 *Ibid*, folder A, address to Annual Missions Conference, November 1954.
12 *Ibid*, draft Annual Report for 1953–54.
13 Elizabeth Burchill, *New Guinea nurse* (Adelaide), 1967, pp. 92–4.
14 Refshauge Papers, draft Annual Report for 1953–54.
15 Refshauge Papers, folder A; address to Annual Mission Conference, 1954.
16 See MHR Tapes 5, 6 and 7, interview with Sister Betty Crouch.
17 Refshauge Papers, draft Annual Report for 1955–56.
18 D. J. van de Kaa, 'The demography of Papua New Guinea's indigenous population', Unpublished PhD thesis, Australian National University, 1971, p. 19.
19 P. Townsend, 'Working towards equality in Family Health Services', Waigani seminar paper, 1982.
20 1981 Papua New Guinea National Census.
21 van de Kaa, 'PNG demography', pp. 63–4.
22 Lea and Lewis, 'Masculinity in Papua New Guinea', pp. 65–78.
23 1981 Papua New Guinea National Census.
24 Young, 'Tropology of the Dobu Mission', pp. 97–100.
25 Michael Young, 'Children's illness and adult's ideology: patterns of health care on Goodenough Island, Milne Bay Province', *PNGMedJ*, 24:3 (1981), 179–87.

26 See the national figures in the *United Nations Demographic Yearbooks*.
27 Barbara D. Miller, *The endangered sex: neglect of female children in rural north India* (Cornell, 1981), pp. 107–32.
28 Paul R. Greenough, *Prosperity and misery in modern Bengal: the famine of 1943–44* (Oxford, 1982), pp. 182–236.

11 Health education

1 Robert Black, 'The health of patrol officers in the Territory of Papua and New Guinea', *MJA*, 2 (1959) 428–35.
2 Dr Martha Macintyre, personal communication, 1985.
3 J. T. Gunther, 'Medical services, history', in *Encyclopaedia of Papua New Guinea*.
4 Margaret Spencer, *Doctor's wife in New Guinea* (Sydney, 1959), pp. 26–7.
5 Gunther, 'Medical services, history'.
6 Radford, 'Papua New Guinea's barefoot doctors', pp. 121–2.
7 Peter Calvert, 'The rural health worker', *PNGMedJ*, 13:1 (1970), 13–17.
8 Ellen Kettle, *That they might live*, pp. 143–6.
9 *Ibid*, p. 143.
10 *Ibid*, pp. 143–8.
11 MHR tapes, 5, 6 and 7.
12 Refshauge Papers, Australian National Library, draft annual report of the MCH Division for 1952–53.
13 MHR tapes, 9 and 10, Sir Cecil Abel and Nedulia.
14 Kettle, *That they might live*, p. 61.
15 Ann Kaniku, 'Milne Bay women', in D. Denoon and R. Lacey (eds.), *Oral tradition in Melanesia* (Port Moresby, 1981), pp. 188–206.
16 Refshauge Papers, draft annual reports from 1952–53 onwards.
17 Marie Reay, 'Women in transitional society', in E. K. Fisk (ed.), *New Guinea on the threshold* (Canberra, 1966), pp. 166–84.
18 Patrick Vaughan, 'The medical assistant in Papua and New Guinea', *PNGMedJ*, 11 (1968), 81–84.
19 *Pacific Islands Monthly*, January 1952.
20 Albert Maori Kiki, *Ten thousand years in a lifetime* (Melbourne, 1968), p. 70.
21 CRS. A518: U 832/1/3, part 3. Gunther to Minister, 6 November 1951.
22 Robert L Pulsford, 'The teaching of the behavioural sciences at the Papuan Medical College', *PNGMedJ*, 11:2 (1968), 67–8.
23 *Ibid*.
24 *Ibid*.
25 *Ibid*.
26 V. Lynn Meek, *The University of Papua New Guinea: a case study in the sociology of higher education* (Brisbane, 1982).
27 G. C. Cook, 'The training of doctors and the delivery of health care in Papua New Guinea'; and J. K. A. Clezy, 'Doctors' dilemma', both in *PNGMedJ*, 22:3 (1979) 163–5, 165–6. See also J. K. A. Clezy, 'Medical education in PNG: 40 years on', in *Niugini Nius*, 25 and 26 July 1986.
28 This judgment is based on nine years of discussion in the Academic Board of the University of Papua New Guinea. See also K. Somers, WHO Consultant's Report on the Faculty of Medicine, UPNG, March 1974.
29 Lyn Calvert, 'Hygiene or habit?' *PNGMedJ*, 13:1 (1970), 17–20.

12 A national health system

1 Radford, 'Papua New Guinea's barefoot doctors', pp. 115–27.
2 Hakan Hellberg, 'Co-ordination of Health Department and church/mission resources', in Bell, *Diseases and health services of PNG*, pp. 572–4.
3 *Ibid.*
4 Peter Smith, 'Education and colonial control: a history of education in Papua New Guinea, 1871–1975', Unpublished PhD thesis, University of Papua New Guinea, 1986.
5 Peter Strang, 'A missionary doctor's disquiet', undated (?1970) roneo, in Dr Strang's papers relating to the Churches Medical Council; later published in *The Missionary Review*, 81:1 (1973), 35–42.
6 Peter Smith, 'Education and political control'.
7 Strang Papers, 'Working together – a review', roneo, occasional paper 2 for the Churches Medical Council, 16 July 1973.
8 Strang Papers, Peter Strang, 'The new commitment in wider service', CMC Occasional Paper No. 1, March 1973.
9 Strang, 'A missionary doctor's disquiet', pp. 35–42.
10 Strang Papers, 'Working together'.
11 For example, Yagaum Lutheran Hospital became a health centre, while Madang General Hospital became the provincial general hospital.
12 J. T. Griffin, 'Cautious deeds and wicked fairies: a decade of independence in Papua New Guinea', *JPH*, 21:4 (1987), 188.
13 Papua New Guinea Government, *1974–78 National Health Plan* (Port Moresby, 1973).
14 PNG Department of Health and National Planning Office, *1983 Health Policy Review*.
15 Griffin, 'Cautious deeds and wicked fairies', pp. 183–201.
16 ed. Clive Bell (Port Moresby, 1973).
17 John Gunther, 'Kuru and a Nobel Prize'.
18 David Turnbull, 'The quest for a malaria vaccine', paper at ANZAAS Congress, Townsville, 1987.
19 See for example the autobiographical information in a series of *PNGMedJ* articles: Andrew J. Hall, 'A provincial health officer in Papua', 25:1 (1982), 50–2; Christopher E. Lennox, 'A Medical Superintendent in the highlands of Papua New Guinea', 25:2 (1982), 127–30; Andrew Tulloch, 'The role of the paediatrician in Papua New Guinea', 25:3 (1982), 182–5; and Peter J. Halstead, 'A District Medical Officer in West New Britain, Papua New Guinea', 25:4 (1982), 273–8.
20 Ken Clezy, 'Medical education in PNG: 40 years on'.
21 J. Richardson, 'Health and health care in Papua New Guinea: problems and solutions', in C. D. Throsby (ed.), *Human resources development in the Pacific* (ANU, Canberra, 1987), pp. 25–52; Stephen Frankel, 'Peripheral health workers are central to primary health care: lessons from Papua New Guinea's aid posts', *Social Science and Medicine*, 19:3 (1984), 279–90, esp. 288–90.

13 Primary health care

1 Scragg, 'Lemankoa', pp. 12–13.
2 e.g. Maddocks, 'Communicable disease in Papua New Guinea', p. 123.
3 Doyal and Pennell, *Political economy of health*, chapter 7.
4 Kingsley Gee, 'Primary health care in Papua New Guinea', *PNGMedJ* 26:3–4

(1983), 168–9. The fullest account of the strategy is in World Health Organisation, *Primary health care: Alma Ata 1978* (Geneva, 1978).

5 Maurice King, *Medical care in developing nations* (Oxford, 1966).

6 *Lancet*, 1 (1972), pp. 679–81.

7 Editorial, *PNGMedJ*, 8:3 December (1965), 69–70.

8 (Cornell, 1969).

9 Ian Maddocks, '*Udumu A-Hagaia*', inaugural lecture, University of Papua New Guinea (Port Moresby, 1971).

10 Editorial, *PNGMedJ*, 9:3 (October 1986), 77–8.

11 See chapter 12.

12 R. F. R. Scragg, 'Specialists and spraymen', *PNGMedJ*, 11:2 (1968), 43–8.

13 J. T. Griffin, 'Cautious deeds and wicked fairies', p. 188.

14 Luise Parsons, 'Aid posts in Enga Province', *PNGMedJ*, 25:3 (1982), 173–5.

15 John Biddulph, 'Legislation to protect breast feeding', *PNGMedJ*, 26:1 (1983), 9–12.

16 Janice Reid, 'The role of Maternal and Child Health Clinics in education and prevention: a case study from Papua New Guinea', in *Social Science and Medicine*, 19:3 (special issue 1984), 291–303.

17 Glen Mola and Iain Aitken, 'Maternal mortality in Papua New Guinea, 1976–1983', *PNGMedJ*, 27:3–4 (1984), 65–72.

18 D. Wohlfahrt and K. Kukyuwa, 'Village rural water supplies in the Western Highlands Province of Papua New Guinea', *PNGMedJ*, 25:3 (1982), 168–72.

19 Editorial *PNGMedJ*, 8:3 (December 1965), 69–70.

20 John Biddulph, 'Doctors in Papua New Guinea – current and future supply', *PNGMedJ*, 26:3–4 (1983), 207–11.

21 Paul Crouch, 'The changing role of the Health Extension Officer in Papua New Guinea', *PNGMedJ*, 25:2 (1982), 77–8.

22 Department of Health and National Planning Office, *1983 Health Policy Review*.

23 *Ibid*.

24 *Ibid* and Gee, 'Primary health care in PNG', pp. 168–9.

25 Papua New Guinea 1981 Census, preliminary report.

26 *Ibid*.

27 John Lourie, 'Editorial: Ok Tedi, pot of what?' in *PNGMedJ*, 26:2 (1983), 91–2; and Peter Heywood, 'Progress report on the 1982/83 national nutrition survey', PNG Institute of Medical Research, Madang, mimeo, 1983.

28 Scragg, 'Lemankoa', *passim*.

29 Taukuro, B. D. *et al.*, 'The World Health Organisation North Fly clinico-epidemiological pilot study, *PNGMedJ*, 23:2 (1980), 80–6.

30 Lourie, 'Ok Tedi: pot of what?'.

31 Julian Tudor Hart, 'The inverse care law', *Lancet*, 1 (1971), 405–12.

32 A. J. Radford, 'The inverse care law in Papua New Guinea', in N. F. Stanley and R. A. Joske (eds.), *Changing disease patterns and human behaviour* (London, 1980), pp. 323–43.

33 Department of Health and NPO, *1983 Health Policy Review*.

34 C. A. Valentine and B. L. Valentine, *Going through changes: villagers, settlers and development in Papua New Guinea* (Port Moresby, 1979), pp. 49–72.

35 Elizabeth Cox, 'Gavien and Bagi: rubber/profit vs people/community' in Valentine and Valentine, *Going through changes*, pp. 15–34.

36 This issue is taken up by Barry Shaw, 'The children of the Kyaka Enga'.

37 Scragg, 'Lemankoa', table 3.5

38 Mola and Aitken, 'Maternal mortality in PNG, 1976–1983', pp. 65–72.

39 *Ibid*; and Martha Macintyre, 'Changing paths'. For an imaginative response to

the general problem, see Peter Barss and Kate McCallum, 'Tubal ligation in Milne Bay Province', *PNGMedJ*, 26:3–4 (1983), 174–7.
40 Robin L. Hide, 'Sex differences in some physical effects of ageing and mortality risk', typescript, 1984.
41 L. A. Malcolm, *Growth and development in New Guinea – a study of the Bundi people of the Madang District* (Goroka, Institute of Human Biology, 1970).
42 Michael Young, '"Our name is women; we are bought with limesticks and limepots": an analysis of the autobiographical narrative of a Kalauna woman', *Man* (NS) 18 (1983), 481.
43 Griffin, 'Cautious deeds and wicked fairies', pp. 186–7.
44 Maddocks, 'Medicine and colonialism', *Australian and New Zealand Journal of Sociology*, 11:3 (1975), 33.
45 Nancy C. Frith, R. G. Hausfeld and P. M. Moodie, *The Coasttown Project: action research in Aboriginal community health*, Australian Department of Health, School of Public Health and Tropical Medicine, service publication XI (Canberra, 1974).

Bibliography

1 Archives: Australian Commonwealth Records Series (CRS)

Department of Territories archives, Mitchell Depository, Commonwealth Archives of Australia, Canberra.

School of Public Health and Tropical Medicine (including Australian Institute of Tropical Medicine), Sydney Depository, Commonwealth Archives of Australia.

Commonwealth Department of Health archives, Mitchell Depository, Commonwealth Archives of Australia, Canberra.

2 Private papers

John Cameron's papers, Department of Pacific and Southeast Asian History, Australian National University.

Brigadier Disher's papers, Melbourne University Archives.

Sir John Gunther's papers, Australian National University Archives.

Dr Norma MacArthur's papers, including reports by Dr Bellamy, in the possession of the author.

Dr Joan Refshauge's papers, Australian National Library, Canberra.

Dr Peter Strang's papers, in the possession of Dr Strang.

3 Records of interview

Medical History Research (MHR) tapes.

Tapes held in the Records Room, Department of Pacific History, Australian National University; and copies in the New Guinea Collection, University of Papua New Guinea Library:

(1) Sister Alexis and Father John Tschauder
(2) Father John Tschauder
(3) Reverend and Mrs K Holzknecht
(4) Reverend and Mrs K Holzknecht and Reverend Gerhardt Reitz
(5) Sister Betty Crouch
(6) Sister Betty Crouch
(7) Sister Betty Crouch
(8) Sister Winifred
(9) Nedulia
(10) Sir Cecil Abel
(11) Hera Ganiga
(12) Edwin Tscharke
(13) Edwin Tscharke
(14) Edwin Tscharke
(15) Edwin Tscharke and Siming Aksim

(16) Cliff Smith
(17) Cliff Smith and Tinsley Health Workers
(18) Tinsley Health Workers
(19) Ester Stotik and Matron Reto
(20) Dr Timothy Pyakalyia and Pakea Rita
(21) Del Weinholdt
(22) Dudley and Marjorie Deasey
(23) Dudley and Marjorie Deasey
(24) Siming Aksim and Fulalek
(25) Sir John Gunther
(26) Sir John Gunther
(27) Sir John Gunther
(28) Sir John Gunther
(29) Sir John Gunther
(30) Sir John Gunther
(31) Peter Calvert
(32) Sister Marie Paul
(33) Archbishop Strong
(34) Percy Chatterton

Interviews were also conducted with Dr Joan Refshauge (by her brother Sir William Refshauge), Sir William Refshauge, Mr Stan Christian, Mr Bert Speer, Mr Keke Mareva, Professor Robert Black, Sir Frank Fenner, Sir Macfarlane Burnet, Professor Kris Somers, Professor Roy Scragg, and Professor Ian Maddocks.

4 Bibliographies

Alpers, M. P., D. C. Gajdusek and S. G. Ono. *Bibliography of Kuru* (Bethseda, Maryland, 1975).
Black, Robert H. *A bibliography of malaria in the South–West Pacific* (Commonwealth Institute of Health, Tropical Medicine Technical Paper VI, Canberra, 1981).
Hornabrook, R. W. and Skeldon, G. H. F. (eds.) *A bibliography of medicine and human biology in Papua New Guinea* (PNG Institute of Medical Research, Faringdon, 1977), and later supplements.
Thompson, A.-G. *The Southwest Pacific: an annotated guide to bibliographies, indexes and collections in Australian libraries* (Canberra, 1986).

5 Government publications

Bell, Clive O. *The diseases and health services of Papua New Guinea* (Department of Public Health, Port Moresby, 1973).
Bell, C. O. 'Organisation and administration of the health services', in Bell, *Diseases and health services of PNG*, pp. 417–25.
Burton-Bradley, B. G. *Longlong! Transcultural psychiatry in Papua and New Guinea* (Department of Public Health, Port Moresby, 1973).
Cilento, Raphael W, *The white man in the tropics* (Commonwealth Department of Health, Tropical Division, Service Publication VII, Melbourne, 1925).
  The causes of the depopulation of the Western Islands of the Territory of New Guinea (Canberra, 1928).
Department of Health. *The story of TB* (Port Moresby, 1963).
German New Guinea Annual Reports (GNGAR). Edited and translated by Peter Sack and Dymphna Clark, (ANU Press, Canberra, 1979).

Hellberg, Hakan. 'Co-ordination of Health Department and church/mission resources', in Bell, *Diseases and health services of PNG*, pp. 572–4.

Hermant, P. and Cilento, Raphael W. *Report of the mission entrusted with a survey on health conditions in the Pacific Islands* (League of Nations Health organisation, Geneva, 1929).

Hipsley, E. H. and F. W. Clements (eds.) *Report of the New Guinea Nutrition Survey Expedition, 1947* (Department of External Territories, Canberra, 1947).

Mandated Territory of New Guinea Annual Reports (NGAR).

Papua New Guinea Department of Health and National Planning Office, *1983 Health Policy Review* (Port Moresby, 1983).

Papua New Guinea Department of Public Health. *Annual Reports: Territory of Papua New Guinea Annual Reports*.

Papua New Guinea Department of Public Health *Tuberculosis in Papua and New Guinea*, by D. Jamieson (Port Moresby, 1955).

Papua New Guinea Government. *The 1974 National Health Plan* (Port Moresby, 1973).

Papuan Annual Reports (PAR).

Parkinson, A. D. and Tavil, N. W. 'Malaria', in Bell, *Diseases and health services of PNG*, pp. 162–78.

Russell, D. A. *Notes on leprosy* (PNG Department of Public Health, 1962).

Russell, D. A. and Bell, C. O. 'Leprosy', in Bell, *Diseases and health services of PNG*, pp. 185–90.

Smith, M. C. Staniforth. *Handbook of the Territory of Papua* (Melbourne, 1907, 1909, 1912; and Canberra, 1927).

Somers, K. *World Health Organisation Consultant's Report on Assistance to Faculty of Medicine, University of Papua New Guinea (1974)*.

Strong, Walter Mersh. *Handbook on the treatment and prevention of disease in Papua, when medical advice is unobtainable* (Port Moresby, 1917, 1926).

Improving the food supplies of native villages (Port Moresby, 1926).

The feeding of native labourers in Papua (Port Moresby, 1926).

Bacillary dysentery (Port Moresby, 1932).

Vitamins (Port Moresby, 1932).

Minor infectious diseases in natives (Port Moresby, 1933).

Wigley, Stan C. 'Tuberculosis', in Bell, *Diseases and health services of PNG*, pp. 179–84.

6 Journals

Journal of Pacific History (JPH)
Lancet
Medical Journal of Australia (MJA)
Papua New Guinea Medical Journal (PNGMedJ)
Territory Health Bulletin

7 Books and Articles

Anon. 'Editorial: man-made malaria', *PNGMedJ* 1:4 (1956), 116.

Anon. [various authors] *The Institute of Medical Research 1900–1950* (Kuala Lumpur, Government Press, 1951).

Anon. '47 Yia bihain', *Wantok*, 31 January 1981.

Anon. 'Training Papuan Medical Assistants', *Pacific Islands Monthly*, 6 (1935), 9.

Anon. 'Editorial: the medical missionary', *PNGMedJ*, 9:4 (1966), 117–8.

Anon (Ian Maddocks). 'Editorial: medical care in developing countries', *PNGMedJ*, 8:3 (1965), 69–70.

'Editorial: has it all been worth while?', *PNGMedJ*, 9:3 (1966), 77–8.

Backhouse, T. C. and E. Ford. 'Obituary: George Aloysius Makinson Heydon', *MJA*, 2 (1963), 465–7.

Balfour, A. and H. H. Scott. *Health problems of the empire: past, present and future* (London, 1924).

Barss, Peter and Kate McCallum, 'Tubal ligation in Milne Bay Province, Papua New Guinea', *PNGMedJ*, 26:3–4 (1983), 174–7.

Bassett, Marnie. *Letters from New Guinea 1921* (Melbourne, 1969).

Benjamin, Amos, and John Biddulph. 'Port Moresby Infant Feeding Survey, 1979', *PNGMedJ.*, 23:2 (1980), 92–6.

Biddulph, John. 'Legislation to protect breast feeding', *PNGMedJ*, 26:1 (1983), 9–12.

'Doctors in Papua New Guinea – current and future supply', *PNGMedJ*, 26:3–4 (1983).

Black, Robert H. 'Malaria control in the Southwest Pacific', *South Pacific*, 8 (1955), 56–61.

'The epidemiology of malaria in the South West Pacific', *South Pacific*, 9:6 (1956), 417–22.

'Dr Bellamy of Papua', three parts, *MJA* 2 (1957), pp. 189–97, 232–8, 279–84.

'Health Education in Papua and New Guinea', *South Pacific*, 10:1 (1958), 1–7.

'The health of patrol officers in the Territory of Papua and New Guinea', *MJA*, 2 (1959), pp. 428–34.

'Health, housing and urban development' *PNGMedJ*, 8:2 (1965), 65–6.

'The role of rural health services in disease eradication programmes', *PNGMedJ*, 13:1 (1970), 7–10.

Browne, S. G. 'Prospects for the control of leprosy in Papua New Guinea', *PNGMedJ*, 26:1 (1983), 1–2.

Buckley, K. and K. Klugman. *The history of Burns Philp, the Australian company in the South Pacific* (Sydney, 1981).

Burchill, Elizabeth. *New Guinea nurse* (Adelaide, 1967).

Burton, John, 'A dysentery epidemic in New Guinea, and its mortality', *JPH*, 28:4 (1983), 236–61.

Butler, A. G. *et al. The Australian Army Medical Services in the War of 1914–1918* (2nd edn, Melbourne, 1938).

Calvert, Lyn. 'Hygiene or habit?' *PNGMedJ* 13:1 (1970), 17–20.

Calvert, Peter. 'The rural health worker', *PNGMedJ* 13:1 (1970), 13–18.

Charlwood, J. D. 'Which way now for malaria control?', *PNGMedJ*, 27:3–4 (1984), 159–62.

Cilento, Raphael W. 'Causes of depopulation among some island people', *MJA*, 2 (1924), 486.

'Food deficiencies in New Guinea, *MJA*, 1 (1926), 309–13.

'Nutrition and numbers', *The Livingstone Lectures 1936*.

'Obituary: J. S. C. Elkington', *MJA*, 2 (1955), 259–60.

Cilento, R. W. and C. Lack. *Triumph in the tropics: an historical sketch of Queensland* (Brisbane, 1959).

Clements, F. W. 'A tuberculosis survey of a Papuan village', *MJA*, 2 (1936), 253–8.

Clezy, Ken. 'A degree course in medicine in Papua and New Guinea', *PNGMedJ*, 8:2 (1965).

'Doctors dilemma', *PNGMedJ*, 22:3 (1979), 165–6.

'Medical education in PNG: 40 years on', two parts, *Niugini Nius*, 25 and 26 July 1986.

Cook, G. C. 'The training of doctors and the delivery of health care in Papua New Guinea', *PNGMedJ*, 22:3 (1979).

Cox, Elizabeth. 'Gavien and Bagi: rubber/profit vs people/community', in Valentine and Valentine, *Going through changes*.

Crane, G. 'Perspectives on the treatment of tropical splenomegaly syndrome', paper presented at the 19th annual symposium of the PNG Medical Society, Lae, 1983.

Crouch, Paul. 'The changing role of the Health Extension Officer in Papua New Guinea', *PNGMedJ*, 25:2 (1982).

Davies, John. 'Medical specialists in Papua New Guinea: the planned use of doctors and allied health workers', *PNGMedJ*, 25:3 (1982).

Denoon, Donald. 'Capitalism in Papua New Guinea', *JPH*, 20:3–4 (1985), 119–34.

'Temperate medicine and settler capitalism: on the reception of western medical ideas', in R. MacLeod (ed.), *Disease, medicine and empire* (Routledge, London, in press), pp. 121–38.

'Walter Mersh Strong', in B. G. Burton-Bradley (ed.), *The history of medicine in Papua New Guinea* (Sydney, in press).

Denoon, Donald and Catherine Snowden. *A time to plant and a time to uproot: a history of agriculture in Papua New Guinea* (Port Moresby, 1981).

Douglas, R. A. 'Dr Anton Breinl and the Australian Institute of Tropical Medicine', three parts. *MJA*, 1 (1977), 713–16, 748–51, 784–90.

Doyal, L., with I. Pennell. *The political economy of health* (London, 1979).

du Toit, B. M. *Akuna: a New Guinea village community* (Rotterdam, 1975).

Earner, Paul. 'Return of an old enemy', *Times of Papua New Guinea*, 6 August 1984.

Ewers, William H. 'Malaria in the early years of German New Guinea', *Journal of the Papua New Guinea Society*, 6 (1973), 3–30.

Firth, Stewart G. *New Guinea under the Germans* (Melbourne, 1983).

'German New Guinea: the archival perspective', *JPH*, 20:1–2 (1985), 94–103.

Fisher, F. G. 'Raphael West Cilento, Medical Administrator, Legislator, and Visionary', unpublished PhD thesis, University of Queensland, 1984.

Fleming Jones, R. 'Tropical diseases in British New Guinea', in *Transactions of the Royal Society for Tropical Medical Hygiene*, 5 (1910–11), 93–105.

Frankel, Stephen. 'Peripheral health workers are central to primary health care: lessons from Papua New Guinea's aid posts', *Social Science and Medicine*, 19:3 (1984), 279–90.

Garruto, Ralph M. 'Disease patterns of isolated groups', in Henry R. Rothschild (ed.), *Biocultural aspects of disease* (New York, 1981), pp. 557–97.

Gee, Kingsley 'Editorial: primary health care in Papua New Guinea', *PNGMedJ*, 26:3–4 (1983), 168–9.

Gillespie, Jim. 'The hookworm campaign and a national health policy in Australia, 1911–1930', ANZAAS Congress paper, Townsville, 1987.

Golson, Jack. 'Agriculture in New Guinea: the long view'; 'Agricultural technology in New Guinea'; and 'New Guinea agricultural history: a case study', in Denoon and Snowden, *A history of agriculture in Papua New Guinea*, pp. 33–42, 43–54, 55–64.

Gordon, D. 'Obituary: Sir Raphael West Cilento', *MJA*, 1 (1985), 144–5.

Grenfell Price, A. 'The white man in the Tropics', *MJA*, 1 (1933), 106–10.

Griffin, J. T. 'Cautious deeds and wicked fairies: a decade of independence in Papua New Guinea', *JPH*, 21:4 (1987), 183–201.

Griffin, J. T., Hank Nelson and S. G. Firth, *Papua New Guinea: a political history* (Melbourne, 1979).

Gunther, Sir John T. 'Kuru and a Nobel Prize', typescript, Department of Pacific & Southeast Asian History, Australian National Univ., n.d.

'Eighty per cent man', typescript, n.d.

'Epidemiology of malaria in Papua New Guinea', *PNGMedJ*, 1:1 (1955), 1–9.

'Obituary: Eric Giblin', *PNGMedJ*, 1:2 (1955), 81.

'Medical services, history', in *Encyclopaedia of Papua New Guinea* (Melbourne, 1972).

'The early history of malaria control in Papua New Guinea', *PNGMedJ*, 17:1 (1974), 4–7.

Hall, Andrew J. 'A provincial health officer in Papua', *PNGMedJ*, 25:1 (1982), 50–2.

Hallpike, C. R. *Bloodshed and vengeance in the Papuan mountains: the generation of conflict in Tauade society* (Oxford, 1977).

Halstead, Peter. 'A District Medical Officer in West New Britain Province, Papua New Guinea', *PNGMedJ*, 25:4 (1982), 273–7.

Harloe, Lyn. 'Anton Breinl and the Australian Institute of Tropical Medicine', ANZAAS Congress paper, Townsville, 1987.

Hasluck, Paul. *A time for building: Australian administration in Papua and New Guinea 1951–1963* (Melbourne, 1976).

Haszler, Charles. 'Dr Theodore George Braun: a biographical note', *PNGMedJ*, 8:3 (1965), 82.

'The New Australian doctors in New Guinea', *PNGMedJ*, 10:2 (1967), 35–41.

Heiser, Victor. *A doctor's odyssey: adventures in forty-five countries* (London, 1936).

Herdt, Gilbert (ed.) *Ritualised homosexuality in Melanesia* (Berkeley and London, 1984).

Hetzel, B. S. and P. O. D. Pharoah (eds.) *Endemic cretinism* (Goroka, 1971).

Heywood, Peter. 'Progress report on the 1982/83 national nutrition survey', PNG Institute of Medical Research, Madang, mimeo, 1983.

Hide, Robin L. 'Sex Differences in some physical effects of ageing and mortality risk: a cross-sectional community study with follow-up in Sinasina, Simbu Province, Papua New Guinea', typescript, 1984.

'On the explanation of early childhood mortality decline in Simbu Province, Papua New Guinea', typescript, 1984.

Hopper, Patricia. 'Kicking out the Hun', Unpublished MA thesis, University of Papua New Guinea, 1980.

Hornabrook, R. W. (ed.). *Essays on Kuru* (Faringdon, 1976).

Hughes, Ian. *New Guinea Stone Age trade* (Canberra, 1977).

Inglis, Amirah. *Karo: the life and fate of a Papuan* (Canberra, 1982).

Jenkins, Carol. 'Indigenous childbirth practices', *PNGMedJ*, 27:2 (1984), 61–4.

'The role of traditional medical practice in Papua New Guinea', *PNGMedJ*, 27:3–4 (1984), 121–2.

Jinks, Brian E. 'Policy, planning and administration in Papua New Guinea, 1942–1952, with special reference to the role of Colonel J. K. Murray', unpublished PhD thesis, University of Sydney, 1975.

'Australia's post-war policy for New Guinea and Papua', *JPH*, 18:1–2 (1982), 86–100.

Joyce, Roger. *Sir William MacGregor* (London, 1971).
Kaniku, Ann. 'Milne Bay women', in D. Denoon and R. Lacey (eds.) *Oral tradition in Melanesia* (Port Moresby, 1981), pp. 188–206.
Kettle, Ellen. *That they might live* (Sydney, 1979).
Kiki, Albert Maori. *Ten thousand years in a lifetime: a New Guinea autobiography* (Melbourne, 1968).
Kunz, E. F. *The intruders: refugee doctors in Australia* (Canberra, 1975).
Lambert, S. M. *A doctor in paradise* (London, 1942).
Langmore, Diana. 'European missionaries in Papua 1884–1914, a group portrait', unpublished PhD thesis, Australian National University, 1981.
    '"Exchanging earth for heaven": death in the Papuan missionfields', *Journal of Religious History*, 14:3 (1985), 383–92.
Latukefu, S. 'Oral history and Pacific Island missionaries', in D. Denoon and R. Lacey (eds.) *Oral tradition in Melanesia* (Port Moresby, 1981), pp. 175–87.
Lea, David A. M. and Laurie H. Lewis. 'Masculinity in Papua New Guinea', in L. A. Kosinski and J. W. Webb (eds.) *Population at Microscale* (New Zealand Geographical Society, Auckland, 1976), pp. 65–78.
Leadley, Alan. 'Effects of Japanese occupation on Tolai people', Unpublished MA thesis, University of Papua New Guinea, 1973.
Lebasi, Biga. 'Curtain falls for Kwato's "iron lady"', *Niugini Nius* 2 August 1985.
Lennox, Christopher E. 'A Medical Superintendent in the highlands of Papua New Guinea', *PNGMedJ*, 25:2 (1982), 127–30.
Limbange, Candy K. 'A study of aid post orderly performance in the Wapi Valley in the Enga Province, Papua New Guinea', *PNGMedJ*, 23:3 (1980), 126–31.
Long, Gavin. *The final campaigns* (vol 7, series 1, of *Australia in the War of 1939–1945*, Canberra, 1963).
Lourie, John. 'Editorial: Ok Tedi, pot of what?' *PNGMedJ* 26:2 (1983), 91–2.
Lourie, John, Tukutau Taufa, Jackie Cattani and Bill Anderson. 'Preliminary results of the Ok Tedi medical survey', paper presented at the 19th annual symposium of the PNG Medical Society, Lae, September 1983.
MacArthur, Norma. 'Isolated populations in enclaves or on small islands', in R. J. May and Hank Nelson (eds.), *Melanesia: beyond diversity* (Canberra, 1982), I, pp. 27–32.
McDowell, Nancy. 'Reproductive decision making and the value of children: the Bun of Angoram District, East Sepik Province', IASER, Port Moresby, 1981.
    'Reproductive decision making and the value of children in rural Papua New Guinea', IASER, Port Moresby, 1981.
MacGregor, Sir William. 'Some problems of tropical medicine', *Lancet*, 13 October 1900, pp. 1055–61.
Macintyre, Martha. 'Changing paths: an historical ethnography of the traders of Tubetube', unpublished PhD thesis, Australian National University, 1983.
MacKenzie, S. S. *The Australians at Rabaul* (4th edn, Sydney, 1937).
MacLaren, H. and Christopher Lennox. 'Child health clinics in Enga Province', *PNGMedJ*, 24, 2 (1981), 99–102.
Maddocks, Ian, 'Has it all been worthwhile?' *PNGMedJ*, 9:3 (1966), 77–8.
    Editorial, *PNGMedJ*, 10:2 (1967), 33–4.
    'Communicable disease in Papua and New Guinea', *PNGMedJ*, 13:4 (1970), 120–4.
    '*Udumu A-Hugaia*' (inaugural lecture, University of Papua New Guinea, 1971).
    'Medicine and colonialism', *Australian and New Zealand Journal of Sociology*, 11:3 (1975).

Maguire, F. A. and R. W. Cilento. 'The occupation of German New Guinea', in Australian War Memorial, Melbourne, *The Australian Army Medical Services in the War of 1914–1918* (2nd edn, Melbourne, 1938).

Malcolm, L. A. *Growth and development in New Guinea – a study of the Bundi people of the Madang District* (Institute of Human Biology, Goroka, Monograph 1, 1970).

Mareva, Keke. 'My struggles for development', typescript in possession of the author, Port Moresby 1981.

May, Robert M. 'Parasitic infections as regulators of animal populations', *American Scientist* 71 (1983), 36–45.

Mayo, John. 'Oddity of empire: British New Guinea 1884–1888', Unpublished MA thesis, University of Papua New Guinea, 1972.

Meek, V. Lynn. *The University of Papua New Guinea: a case study in the sociology of higher education* (Brisbane, 1982).

Miklouho-Maclay, N. N. *Travels to New Guinea: diaries, letters, documents*, compiled and introduced by D. Tumarkin (Moscow, 1982).

Mitchell, William E. 'Culturally contrasting therapeutic systems of the West Sepik: the Lujere', in T. R. Williams (ed.), *Psychological anthropology* (The Hague, 1975), pp. 409–39.

Moi, Wilfred. 'Experiences in psychiatry as a general practitioner in Papua and New Guinea over a period of 15 years', typescript, n.d.

'Life history of Dr Wilfred Keina Moi', typescript, 1983.

Mola, Glen and Iain Aitken. 'Maternal mortality in Papua New Guinea, 1976–1983', *PNGMedJ*, 27:3–4 (1984), 65–72.

Nash, J. 'The role of the Leprosy Mission in the national tuberculosis/leprosy programme', paper at PNG Medical Society 19th Annual Symposium, Lae, 1983.

Nelson, Hank N. 'Brown doctors, white prejudice', *New Guinea*, 5:2 (1970), 21–8.

Black, white and gold: goldmining in Papua New Guinea, 1878–1930 (Canberra, 1976).

'A note on the scale of dying: the Japanese 1942–1945', in R. J. May and Hank Nelson (eds.), *Melanesia: beyond diversity* (Canberra, 1982), pp. 175–8.

Taim Biling Masta: the Australian involvement with Papua New Guinea (Sydney, 1982).

Neumann, Klaus. 'Will the missionary shoot the "smallpox spirit"', seminar paper, Pacific History, Australian National University, 1985.

Oram, Nigel D. 'Health, housing and urban development', *PNGMedJ*, 8:2 (1965), 41–51.

Parkinson, H. R. *Dreissig Jahre in der Südsee* (Stuttgart, 1907).

Parsons, Luise. 'Aid posts in Enga Province', *PNGMedJ*, 25:3 (1982), 173–5.

Pernetta, J. and L. Hill. 'Subsidy cycles in consumer/producer societies: the face of change', in Denoon and Snowden, *A history of agriculture in Papua New Guinea*, pp. 293–309.

Peters, W. 'Malaria control in Papua and New Guinea', *PNGMedJ*, 3:3 (1959), 66–75.

Pulsford, Robert L. 'The teaching of the behavioural sciences at the Papuan Medical College', *PNGMedJ*, 11:2 (1968), 67–8.

Pulsford, R. L., and J. Cawte. *Health in a developing country* (Brisbane, 1972).

Radford, Anthony, J. 'Papua New Guinea's barefoot doctors, the aid post orderly and his predecessor the medical tultul', in H. Attwood and R. W. Home (eds.), *Patients, practitioners and techniques* (Melbourne, 1984), pp. 115–27.

'The inverse care law in Papua New Guinea', in N. F. Stanley and R. A.˙Joske (eds.), *Changing disease patterns and human behaviour* (London, 1980), pp. 323–43.

Radford, Anthony J., H. van Leeuwen and S. H. Christian. 'Social aspects in the changing epidemiology of malaria in the highlands of New Guinea', *Annals of Tropical Medicine and Parasitology*, 70:1 (1976), pp. 11–23.

Radford, Robin. *Highlanders and foreigners in the Upper Ramu: the Kainantu area 1919–1942* (Melbourne, 1987).

Reay, Marie. 'Women in transitional society', in E. K. Fisk (ed.), *New Guinea on the threshold* (Canberra, 1966), pp. 166–84.

Reid, Janice. 'Educating mothers: how effective are MCH clinics?', *PNGMedJ*, 26:1 (1983), 25–8.

'The role of Maternal and Child Health Clinics in education and prevention: a case study from Papua New Guinea', *Social Science and Medicine*, 19:3 (1984), 291–303.

Richardson, J. 'Health and health care in Papua New Guinea: problems and solutions', in C. D. Throsby (ed.), *Human resources development in the Pacific* (ANU, Canberra, 1987), pp. 25–52.

Robinson, Neville K. *Villagers at war: some Papua New Guinea experiences in World War II* (Canberra, 1979).

Rowley, Charles D. 'The promotion of native health in German New Guinea', *South Pacific*, 9:5 (1957), 391–9.

Rudge, G. A. 'Rural health centres', *PNGMedJ*, 6:1 (1962), 33–4.

Ryan, Peter (ed.) *Encyclopaedia of Papua New Guinea* (Melbourne, 1972).

Sack, Peter. 'A history of German New Guinea: a debate about evidence and judgement', *JPH*, 20:1–2 (1985), 84–94.

Schellong, O. 'Die Neu-Guinea-Malaria einst und jetzt', *Archiv für Schiffs–und Tropen-Hygiene*, 5 (1901), 303–27.

Scragg, Roy F. R. 'Depopulation in New Ireland: a study of demography and fertility', unpublished MD thesis, University of Adelaide, 1954.

'Health in the Papua-New Guinea village', *MJA* 1 (1962), 389–95.

'The medical profession in Papua and New Guinea 1884–1984', *Papua New Guinea Scientific Society Annual Report and Proceedings*, 1964, pp. 22–43.

'Specialists and spraymen', *PNGMedJ*, 11:2 (1968).

'Mortality changes in rural New Guinea', *PNGMedJ*, 12:3 (1969), 73–83.

'Lemankoa 1920–1980: a study of the effects of health care intervention', unpublished MA thesis, University of Sydney, 1983.

Sharp, Peter and Philip Harvey. 'Malaria and growth stunting in young children of the highlands of Papua New Guinea', *PNGMedJ*, 23:3 (1980), 132–40.

Shaw, Barry. 'The children of the Kyaka Enga', typescript, Development Studies Centre, Australian National University, 1981.

Skeldon, Ronald (ed.) *The Demography of Papua New Guinea* IASER monograph XI (Port Moresby, 1979).

Smith, Peter. 'Education and colonial control: a history of education in Papua New Guinea, 1871–1975', unpublished PhD thesis, University of Papua New Guinea, 1986.

Snowden, Catherine. 'Copra co-operatives', in Denoon and Snowden, *A history of agriculture in Papua New Guinea*, pp. 185–204.

Southcott, R. V. A. 'Obituary: Charles Mervyn Deland', *MJA*, 2 (1963), 34–5.

Spencer, Margaret. *Doctor's wife in New Guinea* (Sydney, 1959).

John Howard Lidgett Cumpston 1880–1954 (Tenterfield, NSW, 1987).

Stanhope, J. M. 'Patterns of fertility and mortality in rural New Guinea', *New Guinea Research Bulletin*, 34 (Port Moresby, 1970), pp. 24–41.

Strang, Peter J. H. 'A missionary doctor's disquiet', *The Missionary Review*, XXXI, 1 (1973), reprinted in *Catalyst*, 3:4 (1973), 35–42.

'The Church's medical role: the medical missionary in 1974', *Catalyst*, 4:4 (1974), 19–30.

Strong, Walter Mersh. 'Nutritional aspects of depopulation and diseases in the West Pacific, especially in Papua', *MJA*, 2 (1932), 506–12.

'The medical education of Papuan natives', *MJA*, 1 305–9.

'The Health of the People of Papua', *MJA*, 1 (1934), 107–8.

Taukuro, B. D. *et al.* 'The World Health Organisation North Fly clinico-epidemiological pilot study', *PNGMedJ*, 23:2 (1980), 80–6.

Townsend, Patricia K. 'Working towards equality in family health services', Waigani seminar paper, Port Moresby, 1982.

'Infant mortality in the Saniyo-Hiyowe Population, Ambunti District, East Sepik Province', *PNGMedJ*, 28:3 (1985), 177–82.

Tscharke, Edwin G. *A quarter century of healing* (Madang, 1973).

Tulloch, Andrew 'The role of the paediatrician in Papua New Guinea', *PNGMedJ*, 25:3 (1982), 182–5.

Turnbull, David. 'The quest for a malaria vaccine', ANZAAS Congress paper, Townsville, 1987.

Valentine, C. A. and B. L. Valentine (eds.) *Going through changes: villagers, settlers and development in Papua New Guinea* (Port Moresby, 1979).

van de Kaa, D. J. 'The demography of Papua New Guinea's indigenous population', unpublished PhD thesis, Australian National University, 1971.

Vaughan, Berkeley. *Doctor in Papua* (Adelaide, 1974).

Vaughan, Patrick, 'The medical assistant in Papua and New Guinea', *PNGMedJ*, 11:3 (1968), 81–84.

Walker, Allan S. *Clinical problems of war*, Series 5, vol. 1, of *Australia in the War of 1939–1945* (Canberra, 1952).

Middle East and Far East, Series 5, vol. 2 (Canberra 1953).

The island campaigns, Series 5, vol. 3 (Canberra, 1957).

et al. Medical Services of the RAN and RAAF, Series 5, vol. 4 (Canberra, 1961).

Wallace, W. H. *The Wallace story* (Melbourne, n.d., ? 1972).

West, Francis. *Selected letters of Hubert Murray* (Melbourne, 1970).

Whittaker, J. K., N. G. Gash, J. F. Hookey and R. J. Lacey (eds.) *Documents and readings in New Guinea history: prehistory to 1889* (Brisbane, 1975).

Wigley, Stan, 'Tuberculosis and New Guinea: historical perspectives with special reference to the years from 1871 to 1973' in B. G. Burton-Bradley (ed.) *The history of medicine in Papua New Guinea* (Sydney, in press).

Wohlfahrt, D. and K. Kukyuwa, 'Village rural water supplies in the Western Highlands Province of Papua New Guinea', *PNGMedJ*, 25:3 (1982), 168–72.

Young, Michael W. 'A tropology of the Dobu Mission', *Canberra Anthropology*, 3 (1980), 86–104.

'Children's illness and adults' ideology: patterns of health care on Goodenough Island, Milne Bay Province', *PNGMedJ*, 24:3 (1981), 179–87.

'"Our name is women: we are bought with limesticks and limepots"': an analysis of the autobiographical narrative of a Kalauna woman', *Man* (NS) 18 (1983), 478–500.

'Suffer the children: Wesleyans in the D'Entrecasteux', in Margaret Jolly and Martha Macintyre (eds.), *Family and gender in the Pacific: domestic contradictions and the colonial impact* (Cambridge, 1988).

8 Books and Articles on Comparative Topics

Brown, E. R. *Rockefeller medicine men: medicine and capitalism in America* (Berkeley, 1979).

Bryant, J. *Health and the developing world* (Cornell, 1969).

Chen, Lincoln, Emdadul Huq and Stan D'Souza. 'Sex bias in the family allocation of food and health care in rural Bangladesh', *Population and Development Review*, 7:1 (1981), 55–70.

Cummins, C. J. *A history of medical administration in New South Wales 1788–1973* (Sydney, 1979).

Cumpston, J. H. L. *Health and disease in Australia* (ed. and introduced by Milton Lewis) in preparation for publication.

Curtin, Philip D. 'Medical knowledge and urban planning in tropical Africa', *American Historical Review*, 90:3 (1985), 594–613.

Frith, Nancy C., R. G. Hausfeld and P. M. Moodie. *The Coasttown Project: action research in Aboriginal community health*, Australian Department of Health, School of Public Health and Tropical Medicine, Sydney, service publication XI (Canberra 1974).

Goldsmith, J. 'The necessity for the study of tropical medicine in Australia', *Transactions of the Intercolonial Medical Congress* (Hobart 1902), pp. 178–82.

Greenough, Paul R. *Prosperity and misery in modern Bengal: the famine of 1943–44* (Oxford, 1982).

Hart, Julian Tudor. 'The inverse care law', *Lancet*, 1 (1971), 405–12.

Hicks, Neville. *'This sin and scandal': Australia's population debate 1891–1911* (Canberra, 1978).

King, Maurice. *Medical care in developing nations* (Oxford, 1966).

'Medicine in red and blue', *Lancet*, 1 (1972), 679–81.

Logan, J. A. *The Sardinian Project* (Baltimore, 1953).

McArthur, Norma. *New Hebrides population 1840–1967: a reinterpretation* (South Pacific Commission Occasional Paper 18, Noumea, 1981).

Miller, Barbara D. *The endangered sex: neglect of female children in rural north India* (Cornell, 1981).

Olssen, Erik. 'Truby King and the Plunket Society: an analysis of a prescriptive ideology', *New Zealand Journal of History* 15:1 (1981), 3–23.

Oram, Nigel D. 'The growth of towns and separation of racial communities in Uganda', seminar paper, Nuffield College, Oxford, 1960.

Pensabene, T. S. *The rise of the medical practitioner in Victoria* (Canberra, 1980).

Rogers, Barbara. *White health and black poverty* (London, 1976).

Rosen, George. 'Economic and social policy in the development of public health: an essay in interpretation', *Journal of History of Medicine and Allied Sciences*, 8 (1953).

Smith, F. B. *The people's health, 1830–1910* (Canberra, 1979).

Swanson, Maynard. W. 'The sanitation syndrome: bubonic plague and urban native policy in the Cape Colony, 1900–1909', *Journal of African History*, 18:3 (1977), 387–410.

Waksman, S. A. *The conquest of tuberculosis* (Berkeley and Los Angeles, 1966).

Willis, Evan. *Medical dominance: the division of labour in Australian health care* (Sydney, 1983).

Worboys, Michael. 'The emergence of tropical medicine: a study in the establishment of a scientific speciality', in G. LeMaine, R. MacLeod *et al.* (eds.),

Perspectives on the emergence of scientific disciplines (The Hague, 1976), pp. 75–98.

World Health Organisation. *Primary health care: Alma Ata 1978* (Geneva, 1978).

Apartheid and health (Geneva, 1983).

Index